FIT HAPPENS

FIT

HAPPENS

**STRATEGIES FOR LIVING A
HEALTHIER, HAPPIER, FITTER LIFE**

· ·

Joanie
Greggains

· ·

WITH **PATRICIA ROMANOWSKI**

· ·

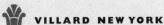 VILLARD NEW YORK

TO MY HUSBAND,

ROBERT McDONALD

Copyright © 2000 by Joanie Greggains

All rights reserved under International and Pan-American Copyright
Conventions. Published in the United States by Villard Books, a division of Random House, Inc., New York, and simultaneously in Canada
by Random House of Canada Limited, Toronto.

Villard Books and colophon are registered trademarks of Random
House, Inc.

Library of Congress Cataloging-in-Publication Data

Greggains, Joanie.
    Fit happens: strategies for living a healthier, happier, fitter
life / Joanie Greggains, with Patricia Romanowski.
        p.   cm.
    ISBN 0-375-50036-7
    1. Health. 2. Nutrition. 3. Physical fitness. I. Romanowski,
Patricia. II. Title.
RA776.G82   1999
613.7—dc21   99-29812

Printed in the United States of America on acid-free paper
Random House website address: www.atrandom.com

98765432

First Edition

Book Design by Barbara M. Bachman

No one truly writes a book alone. I'd like to thank the following people for the support, encouragement, and advice that made this book possible.

In the beginning, Suzanne Wickham Beaird, Random House West Coast Publicity Director, made it all happen. My coauthor, Patty Romanowski, took mounds of information, shaped it, organized it, slapped it, and gave it life. And Lee Boudreaux, our editor at Villard, came at the end of a long line of editors and brought the enthusiasm and evenhanded editorial vision every writer should have. I'd also like to acknowledge the contributions of other Villard editorial staff who preceded her, Annik La Farge and Mollie Doyle.

My assistant, Cindy Renshaw, was, as always, invaluable. Without her, nothing I do would ever get done.

Thank you to Jeannette Boudreau, Esq., Bill Kirby, and Sylvie DeSegur for their professional help, and to my mentors, Philip Dubrow (both in business and in life) and Jim Dunbar (best broadcaster and Renaissance man).

For their professional guidance, I'd like to acknowledge Dr. Arthur White (my friend who always motivates me to reach higher), Dr. Donald Chu, Dr. George Markle, Dr. Brunno Ristow, Dr. Laurie Green, Ann Louise Gittleman, M.S., C.N.S., Dr. Karl Knopf, Paul Yazolino, Dr. Andrew Barnett, Dr. Andrew Carver, Deborah Francesconi, R.N., Shirley Gerrior, Dr. Ronald Smialowicz, JoAnn Tatum Hattner, M.P.H., R.D., Monika, Antony Rivera, and Maury Povich. My coauthor, Patty Romanowski, would like to thank her husband, Philip Bashe, their son, Justin, and her agent, Sarah Lazin, for sticking by through the three years it took us to complete this project.

Very special thanks to my best friend and the best personal trainer, Mary Sherman; my very special girlfriends Melanie Morgan and Patty Garrett; Dallas, the best limousine driver, a great cook, and friend; Joan and Frank Cresci; Robert and Margrit Mondavi; Jack and Elaine LaLanne; Sheila Collins (the Godmother); Sean Galvin (my friend through thick and thin). And for all their help and support, my brother, Ed Ferro, and my sister-in-law, Julie Ferro.

Last but not least, I'd like to acknowledge the memory of my beloved father, Joseph Ferro, and Chuck the Wonder Dog.

Contents

Introduction

How Fit Happens

If you're like most people I know and work with, you see yourself falling into one of two clearly defined camps: those who are fit, healthy, and energetic and those who are out of shape, never quite feeling their best, and perpetually tired. You may have picked up this book because you fall within that second group. Whether this is your first attempt to change how you look and feel or your fifty-first, you may well be thinking, "This time, I'm going to do it"—until you remind yourself—"unless, of course, I give up, like I always seem to do."

Why do we think like this? Why is it that we can run a business, manage a household, and raise a family, yet find ourselves bewildered when it comes to learning how our bodies work and what we can do to stay healthy through our lives? Chances are, you're interested in health and fitness, yet everything you hear—from the latest academic studies to the newest exercise or diet fad—seems to contradict everything else. One hundred people may have one hundred different ideas about the "best" way to eat, the "best" way to exercise, but the one thing I'll bet you all have in common is the idea that fitness is easier for some of us than for others. We tend to believe there's some mystical, unknowable secret that explains how some people keep their weight in a healthy range, exercise regularly and happily, and have the upper hand in their relationship with food. The more we struggle with these problems, the more elusive the solution seems to be.

But here's the secret: There is no secret. When you follow just a few basic principles, fit happens. In the years I've been teaching health and fitness, I've found that people stick to a healthy lifestyle because they've found ways to do it and enjoy it. They have kept or—more likely if they're older—rediscovered the fun in movement, the joy of feeling energetic and alive. Chances are, if you're a veteran of yo-yo dieting, food fads, and exercise gimmicks, you've lost that joy. Because without knowing it, you've been fighting a battle that was lost before it began. Why? Because barring being faced with a question of life or death, human beings simply are not wired to do what they do not enjoy. At first, we can energize and motivate ourselves with the hope of change—or the threat of consequences if we do not. And that can carry us through a new diet or a new exercise regimen, but only for so long. Maybe when you were younger, you could be convinced that carob was "as satisfying as chocolate," and that a boring daily workout was "fun." But you know better now.

Now you need to find the exercise program that is fun for you, the foods you can enjoy without feeling deprived, and a new way to understand and respect your body. Think back to your childhood and how freely and easily you moved through your days—running down a street, chasing your friends in a game of tag, bicycling around the neighborhood, jumping rope, climbing all over the playground, roller skating, jumping on your bed. We moved then because we didn't need to intellectually analyze why we should—we just wanted to. Recapture that spirit and get moving, and you've done the single best thing you can do for yourself. In terms of both long- and short-term health benefits, there is simply no substitute for regular physical exercise. And there is no hope of ever finding a place for exercise in your life if you don't find something you enjoy. Further proof that your inner child can help you achieve the body that will carry you through middle age and beyond can be found in elite fitness centers across the country. They're breaking out the hula hoops and mini trampolines, reviewing the rules of kickball, dodgeball, and relay races. When you make exercise fun, fit can't help but happen.

It seems so simple. How did we miss it before? When it comes to diet, health, and nutrition, we are living in a golden age. Never before in history have we had so much power to improve and lengthen our lives. We have unlocked the secrets of human biology to reveal what our bodies need to function optimally and how to get it. We have devised ways to improve our diets either by enriching them with additives or dietary supplements or by "reengineering" our foods to eliminate unwanted fat, sodium, and sugar. Thousands of years from now, when future archeologists start sifting through skyscraping towers of ancient books about "new" diets and fitness philosophies, miles of videotaped tributes to "unbelievable" and "amazing" exercise apparatus and other allegedly health-enhancing products, what will they think? They might assume that the late-twentieth-century American was as wise, prudent, health conscious, and healthy a specimen of humanity as ever walked—or jogged—the earth. But we Americans are fatter and more out of shape now than at any time in our history, fatter than any civilized country in the world—that's right, the world! And we're not only literally killing ourselves with this inexplicable neglect. We're dooming our children to a life of compromised health and well-being through the poor example we set every day and our lack of vigilance about how badly they eat and how little they exercise. You may not have needed to look beyond your mirror or your window to discover what a recent Harris poll confirmed: 71 percent of Americans age twenty-five and older are overweight. A decade ago—when we were all presumably less health conscious than we are today—only 59 percent of us were in such bad shape. What's happening to us?

Experts have measured it down to the calorie, and it's clear that we move less and eat more than at any time in history. But there's a lot more to the mystery than just that. Why do we opt not to get out and take a brief, invigorating walk? Or take a turn at the kids' hopscotch or a few minutes with a jump rope? Why do we crave foods we know we don't need? Most people's lifestyle is best, and most charitably, described as sedentary. You're probably sitting right now! It's ironic that our kids today clamor for the expensive sneakers and other sports clothing endorsed by their sports heroes, only to wear them to hang out at the mall or sit in front of a computer or television screen. The effort we envision putting forth to change our and our families' habits seems far beyond us, doomed to fail.

But take a minute and ask yourself, "How do I feel right now?" Today it's the fashion to blame low energy levels, an unhealthy lifestyle, and general sense of stress on the demands of our hectic daily lives. We don't have the time, the energy, or the heart to even try this week's new diet or food fad, much less stick with it. An estimated 85 percent of dieters regain the lost weight within two years, and it seems that millions of us have concluded that it's pointless. A 1996 survey found that 20 percent fewer men and 25 percent fewer women said they had dieted in the last six months compared to a 1986 survey. And despite concerns about eating disorders among young women, the number of eighteen- to twenty-four-year-old women who said they were dieting in 1996 was only two thirds what it was a decade before.

We're wary of new health "findings," and with good reason: Even legitimate, well-balanced studies are often misconstrued or distorted by the media. A promising finding that requires further study will be reduced to a headline shouting "Cure!" Worse, though, most of what's touted through books and the media is based on incomplete information or junk science. At the other end of the spectrum are massive tomes dedicated to just one small aspect of a healthy lifestyle. Do any of us really have time to read—and digest—an entire three-hundred-page book on why we shouldn't eat too much fat or how to walk for health? The diet regimens, exercise equipment, drugs, herbs, supplements, vitamins, and their promoters that line the road to good health have turned it from a path paved with common sense to a carnival side show, an endless whirl through a house of mirrors (and isn't that hell?). Logically speaking, little of it makes sense, and we know from experience that the fixes are illusory and temporary. We know diets fail. We know that no additive-infested phony-food diet "dessert product" or diet soft drink will satisfy us or curb our appetite for the real thing. We know that the New Year's resolution to exercise an hour a day from now until the end of time will be forgotten by Valentine's Day (and since the pounds are creeping back anyway, why not have that tenth Godiva truffle?). We know all this, when we should know better.

Why do we fall for it? In most cases, we've never learned enough about how our bodies really work to judge fact from fiction.

If you don't know that all calories count, you may be a victim of the "no fat, no fear" contingent, scrupulously ingesting low- and no-fat foods with the mistaken belief that only fat calories "count."

If you don't understand the basic biology behind food cravings and that afternoon energy slump, you're picking yourself up with coffee and sugar-loaded snacks instead of drinking a tall glass of water and indulging in a two-minute stretch.

If you've been brainwashed into believing that "natural" vitamins are superior to others, that there's really such a thing as "spot reducing," or that any pill or powder can blast, block, or melt away fat, you're throwing away not only money but the precious time you could be using to do something that really works.

You'd think we'd all get the message by now. And judging from the number of us who've lost the will to fight and just succumbed to chronic exhaustion, a sedentary lifestyle—and the extra pounds that come with it—and a sense of personal failure, we get it, all right. Fewer people diet now than ever. What do we learn except how to fail? But here's the best-kept secret in the world: The diets, the fat-erasing supplements, the equipment and paraphernalia fail because they were never meant to work to begin with. If you took the profit motive out of the health- and fitness-related industries, you'd never have heard the words *SnackWell's, NutraSweet, Thighmaster,* or *Beverly Hills Diet.* Have you ever known anyone who "lost 20 pounds in one week" or got "thin thighs in four days"? Unfortunately, the misguided quest for the elusive quick fix dogs most of us from our teens. Binge eating—which is surprisingly common—is now officially recognized as a serious eating disorder, along with anorexia and bulimia. Now even kindergartners are obsessing about their "weight." And it gets even worse. Across the country, school districts are reducing or eliminating physical education from our children's curriculums, and in some places, even canceling recess.

It's time to stop believing and start really knowing, time to start incorporating new health habits that really work and to understand why they do. Every suggestion in this book is geared to teaching you how to eat better, move better, and feel better. Weight loss and a great-looking body—not to mention feeling calmer, less stressed, and more energetic—naturally follow.

I have been teaching people about health and fitness since 1972, when I became a junior high school physical education teacher in the San Francisco public school system. Whether I am hosting my own radio talk show, speaking at a seminar, producing fitness videos, teaching classes, or working with private students at my gym, my goal has never changed. I want to teach you how to understand and respect your body. In doing that, I've developed a very good idea of not only what people *want* to know but also what confuses them and exactly what they *need* to know. This book does not claim to offer everything there is to know. But it is a carefully chosen distillation of all the information you need to know to move toward better health.

Fitness isn't a job or an obligation, it's the natural result of making good, positive lifestyle choices every day. Whether you start with something as simple as making sure you drink enough water or embark on a major daily exercise program, every step counts. Don't wait to reward yourself after you've lost 20 pounds. Give yourself the thumbs up each time you choose to ride your bike instead of taking the car, each time you bypass the candy machine for the water cooler. Remember, it wasn't one thing you did that got you to where you are today—it was a chain of decisions and events that made it impossible for fit to happen in your life. Substitute smart choices for bad habits and you'll be clearing the way for fit to happen. And, most important, keep it fun. Instead of just exercising, actively pursue the joy in movement you knew as a child. Create a healthy lifestyle from the things you love, and it will last a lifetime.

FIT HAPPENS

Getting Started

1.

I first began working with Rosemary when she was in her late twenties. She had married young, and had two children, ages nine and ten. Within a few minutes of talking to her, I could see that Rosemary was a friendly, caring, and very giving woman. And yet she seemed unhappy. She explained to me how she'd gradually put on 40 pounds in less than a decade, and how she could never say no to anyone. "If someone had a birthday, a baby, a promotion—you name it—I'm the one who offered to get the cake and plan the party. When it came to packing their kids' lunch for school, the other mothers on my block would throw a Lunchables in their backpack and call it a day. Not me. I had to prepare a special egg salad the night before so it would be nicely chilled by morning, then pack it just so because it was for my kids. I baked cookies for my husband's office parties; I volunteered for everything and anything I could. I guess I was just trying to make sure that people liked me. And you know what? I was miserable."

The turning point for Rosemary came one day at work when, as she described it, "One of my coworkers asked me to pick up one party cake too many. I don't know what came over me. I started screaming that I'd had it and who did they think I was: the class mother? Then I drove home fuming, and before dinner announced to my family that I was not going to pack everyone's lunches, and that I wanted more help around the house. When I got done, my husband and my two kids just said, 'Okay, Mom.' I couldn't believe how easy it was."

Rosemary came to me because she was ready to change. Now that she had finally given herself permission to do something for herself, she was going to go all the way. After a brief period of moderate aerobics classes and strength training, she surprised everyone by getting into extreme boot camp–style, high-intensity workouts and the occasional extreme sports weekend. Curious, I asked her why.

"I needed to confront my fears. I used to feel like such a weakling. Now I don't."

LEARN TO LOVE YOUR BODY TO HEALTH

In all the years I've been teaching about fitness and nutrition, I've noticed that most people have at least a general idea of what they would like to achieve in these areas, and why. People's reasons for embarking on a course of change range from the mundane to the inspired. I've worked with people who wanted only to lose a few pounds, and I've worked with people, who, like Rosemary, wanted to find a new life. Through the thousands of people I speak with each year on my radio program and at events, I know that those who try to make the change to health don't always succeed. They start out energized and committed. For several weeks, maybe even a couple of months, things go well enough. But sooner or later—and it's usually sooner—something happens. Weeks will have passed since they hit the gym, rode a bicycle, ate well, or felt up to facing the day.

Experts have lots of theories about why so many of us just give up, and we usually say we "gave up on exercise" or "gave up on trying to lose weight." The real truth, though, is that we give up on ourselves. You can read every diet book ever published, try every exercise regimen known to man. If you don't truly believe that you and your body deserve the best care, the best chance to live long, strong, healthy lives, none of it will matter. You have to learn to love yourself to health.

Don't turn the page until you've read the following list. Put a bookmark right here, because you may find yourself turning back to it—maybe once, maybe twice, maybe every day for the next year. Whenever you need to remind yourself that you do matter, that you do deserve the best physical health, come back to this list.

- **START THINKING ABOUT YOURSELF RATHER THAN THE WORLD OUTSIDE.** Taking control of your health is strictly between you and you. Yes, we are often "prompted" to make changes because our mate would prefer we look "better" or have more energy. And all our friends are constantly dieting and working out. But right now, none of that matters. What matters is what *you* want, and what you are willing to do for *yourself*—not for your friends, your mate, or your dress size.

- **LISTEN TO YOURSELF ONLY WHEN YOU HAVE SOMETHING POSITIVE TO SAY ABOUT YOU.** How many times did your mother say, "If you can't say something nice about somebody, don't say anything at all"? When you hear those nagging, negative self-criticisms start to play in your mind, refuse to listen.

- **REMIND YOURSELF THAT THERE'S MORE TO YOU THAN YOUR BODY.** It sounds obvious, but we often act as if our self-esteem is a stock that rises and falls with the numbers on the scale, or fluctuates with our jeans size or the percentage of fat in last night's dessert. Stop. Even good people eat too much chocolate mousse. (And if *that* was all evil consisted of, what a wonderful world this would be!)

- **TAKE A GOOD LOOK AT YOURSELF** in a full-length mirror, preferably in the privacy of your own home (not in a department store when you're trying on swimsuits). No matter how heavy or how out of shape you are, you are beautiful.

Even if you feel that you are not perfect (and, remember, the best that any of us—and this includes supermodels—can do is create the illusion of perfection), you have features that are unique and attractive: great skin, shiny hair, or shapely legs, for instance.

- **REMEMBER ALL THAT YOUR BODY DOES FOR YOU, AND HONOR IT.** Turn your thinking around. We all know there's room for improvement, but that said, let's look at what your body—even with all its flaws and shortcomings—has done for you. Despite everything good that you may have neglected to do, your body's probably still trying to do the best it can. It takes a lot of abuse to make a body cry "Uncle!" Thank your body for sticking with you, and promise to treat it better from today forward.

- **COMPARE YOURSELF TO PEOPLE WHO REALLY EXIST,** not people you see in movies, on television, or in magazines. It takes a cast of dozens to erect and decorate the cosmetic façade that "civilians" like us accept as a "real" person's face or body. Even the most "natural looking" person you see in the media is the product of expert makeup, hairdressing, costuming, photography, and—often—extensive photo retouching. Believe me, if you had a small "beauty army" at your command, you would look every bit as great.

- **ACCEPT—AND BELIEVE—COMPLIMENTS WHEN YOU RECEIVE THEM.** If someone takes the time to pay you a compliment, accept it graciously and believe it. A compliment is a gift; don't "return" it with self-effacing denials.

- **GIVE YOUR POSITIVE MOVES A POSITIVE SPIN.** The dieter as a martyr is a dangerous, self-defeating stereotype many of us play into. It's okay to feel deprived now and then. But a pervasive air of, "Oh, look how I'm suffering to lose weight and take better care of myself"—which well-meaning loved ones and friends often reinforce—is disingenuous and self-defeating. For one thing, it totally overlooks why you're trying to change your health habits: *You* don't like the way you feel, *you* are not happy with how much you weigh, or *you* are tired of seeing how out of shape you've let yourself get. You can't take responsibility for your future health until you own up to your past and take responsibility for the choices you're making today. When you decline the cheesecake, don't say, "I'm on a diet," the way a tardy teenager would say, "I have to stay for detention." Remember: Whatever sacrifices you may be making toward your goals are ones you've chosen. Somewhere in your heart you believe that you deserve something better from life. If you feel you're being punished, you'll never succeed. But if you embarked on this course for the right reasons—reasons you believe in—stand up for yourself. Unless someone asks, "Why not?" a simple, "No, thank you," will suffice. And if someone does ask or try to persuade you to indulge, say, "I've really cut down on sweets and I feel great, so no, thanks."

IT'S ALL ABOUT HEALTH

When it comes to the thousands of things you can do to improve your health, nothing stands alone. There is no one food, one exercise, one supplement, or one "trick" that will change your life, prevent disease, or give you energy. Changing how you approach your body is no small feat. It seems when we don't get the recognition and support we need as we're trying to change, the road to health begins to feel like a very lonely place. When that happens, I've seen people either quit or opt for the exotic diet or junk-science program, all out of a need to feel that their efforts are being rewarded or that they'll have an edge on the competition at the gym tomorrow or on disease and disability a few decades hence.

Before you come to that fork in the road, I want you to remember this: The "magic formula" to living healthier today and tomorrow is already here. You can't find it in the health food store, your local weight-loss mill, or the noisiest infomercial. And it couldn't be simpler: Eating a good diet, exercising regularly, and maintaining a healthy weight for your body type is really all you need to do to look and feel great. Decades of research, thousands of studies, and the statistics bear out this basic truth too.

Diet and Disease

It's no coincidence that these same diet and fitness recommendations can significantly reduce your risk of developing either of our nation's two biggest killers—heart disease and cancer.

- At least one third and possibly as many as 40 percent of cancers in men and 60 percent of cancers in women may be related to diet.

- A 1995 study found that over 50,000 heart-attack deaths a year could be prevented by simply getting enough folic acid in the diet.

- More early deaths—perhaps as many as 300,000—are caused by diseases related to obesity than by drug abuse or AIDS.

- An estimated 80 percent of all diabetes cases could be prevented simply by eliminating obesity through exercise and diet.

- Sufficient intake of calcium and related minerals and vitamins could reduce the number of potentially deadly hip fractures by 40,000 to 50,000 cases a year.

It's no coincidence that these same lifestyle changes are now recognized as having the potential to alleviate or prevent a long list of conditions, including premenstrual syndrome, osteoarthritis, kidney disease, and osteoporosis. Even if you're in good health, following these principles will make you feel better, work smarter, and live your life more fully.

It's amazing, isn't it? But it shouldn't be. Feeling exhausted every morning, gaining a few pounds every year, and having a hard time getting into the exercise habit are typical of our time; it seems as though almost everyone we know is having the same experience. But you don't need some exotic, restrictive dietary regimen or punishing physical-fitness routine to discover what it really feels like to be alive. It's this simple:

Eat right. Both the American Heart Association and the American Cancer Society endorse these recommendations:

- Limit your total fat intake to 25 percent to 30 percent of your calories. Strive to make at least half of that come from monounsaturated fats (such as olive oil), and split the difference between polyunsaturated fats (no more than 10 percent) and saturated fats (ideally 7 percent and no more than 10 percent). Avoid trans fat. (For more on fat, see "Fat: Unlocking the Right Combination," page 141.)

- Get 55 percent to 60 percent of your calories from complex carbohydrates such as fruits, vegetables, whole-grain products, nuts, seeds, and legumes. Reduce your intake of simple carbohydrates such as desserts, cakes, cookies, pies, soft drinks, and unfortified juices.

- Make sure you're getting your fiber. About 20 to 25 grams a day (not more than 35 grams) may contribute to preventing a range of diseases, specifically colorectal cancer, the second-deadliest cancer (lung cancer is number one), and, according to American Cancer Society estimates for 1998, 29 percent more people die of colorectal cancer than of breast cancer.

- Limit your protein consumption to two to three servings daily of meat, poultry, fish, nuts, and eggs. And make sure you're eating the right-size portion. It's much smaller than you think. (See "Serve Yourself Right: Learn to Size Up a Serving," page 127.)

- Limit your sodium intake to about a teaspoon a day.

Exercise. Contrary to popular belief, the obesity epidemic that's sweeping this country doesn't stem from a huge increase in calories consumed, but from a lack of activity. Exercise does more than just keep you in shape. Exercise can reduce the risks of heart disease, stroke, some forms of cancer, and diabetes. It builds bone mass to withstand osteoporosis, it eliminates the physical damage of stress, and it revitalizes you. Whatever activity you pursue, just get moving for at least half an hour every day.

Don't let your lifestyle ruin your life. Don't smoke and don't drink excessively.

ANOTHER REASON TO FLOSS

To the long list of reasons to floss, add this: It may protect your heart. Flossing prevents gum disease, and though doctors aren't sure exactly why, having gum disease doubles your chances of developing heart disease. More than most other parts of the body, the mouth is dense with blood vessels. One theory is that bacteria get carried through the bloodstream where they can prompt the formation of blood clots, which cause heart attacks.

FOURTEEN WAYS YOUR BODY MAY BE TRYING TO TELL YOU TO EAT BETTER

For all that we hear and read the phrase *listening to our body,* most of us don't do it until it's too late and we can't ignore it. But there's a wide berth—and countless opportunities to improve your health—between now and that future trip to the doctor's office. Of course, any persistent symptom should be checked out by your doctor. Here's a list of common health problems, their nutritional roots, and some possible solutions.

SYMPTOM	CAN BE CAUSED BY	CAN BE ALLEVIATED BY
bad breath	• garlic • onions • fish • cream and other high-fat dairy products • coffee • alcohol	• cutting down on offending foods and drinks • using low-fat and nonfat dairy products • eating parsley
breast tenderness, periodic	• caffeine and methylxanthines in chocolate, coffee, tea, and cola, including decaffeinated versions • water retention • dairy products	• avoiding caffeine and methylxanthine and/or dairy products • increasing your intake of vitamins B_6 and E through supplements or foods • drinking sufficient quantities of water to break the retention cycle (see "The Real Water Cure," page 22)
constipation	• dairy products • too little fiber • not enough water	• eating fewer dairy products • eating more fiber: bran, fruits (especially prunes, figs, and dates), vegetables, and whole-grain breads • drinking at least 8 glasses of water a day
cramps	• insufficient calcium • low consumption of omega-3 fatty acids	• getting 1,200 mg. calcium daily • adding an additional 300 mg. calcium during the first days of your menstrual period • helping your body use the calcium more efficiently by eating high-

SYMPTOM	CAN BE CAUSED BY	CAN BE ALLEVIATED BY *(continued)*
		magnesium foods (whole grains, nuts, leafy green vegetables, and beans) • increasing your omega-3 intake with salmon, tuna, whitefish, sturgeon, mackerel, mullet, herring, bluefish, and anchovies
diarrhea	• too much sorbitol, an ingredient in sugarless gums, candies, and diet sodas • excessive consumption of fruits, vegetables, and bran	• eating a bland diet: bananas, rice, applesauce, and toast (b.r.a.t.)
gas	• eating sorbitol • eating broccoli, brussels sprouts, beans, cabbage, cauliflower, and onions • carbonated drinks • dairy products (if you are lactose-intolerant)	• eating garlic, ginger, or peppermint, which relax a valve in your stomach so that gas passes in burps • avoiding dairy products or eating reduced-lactose or lactose-free foods
hair loss	• crash dieting • excessive amounts of vitamin A, from supplements, liver, and fish oil	• eating a sufficient number of calories • switching to a nontoxic form of vitamin A, found in foods high in beta-carotene (carrots, sweet potatoes, cantaloupe, spinach, broccoli, yellow vegetables, and dried apricots)
headache	• feta cheese, aged cheeses, cured or smoked meats, chicken liver, red wine, chocolate, milk, legumes, coffee, and tea	• eliminating the offending foods

SYMPTOM	CAN BE CAUSED BY	CAN BE ALLEVIATED BY (continued)
	• food additives such as aspartame, monosodium glutamate, and nitrates	
heartburn	• spicy foods, highly acidic foods, and fatty foods • chocolate • alcohol • overeating	• eating a small amount of something else, if you're not too full • trying to eat smaller meals • not sitting or lying down right after eating
hives	• milk, eggs, shellfish, fish, peanuts, berries, or any products made with them • avocados, potatoes, bananas, kiwis, chestnuts, tomatoes, or any products made with them • food additives, such as monosodium glutamate and aspartame	• avoiding these foods (Note: If you experience difficulty breathing, rapid or irregular heartbeat, nausea, diarrhea, fainting, or swelling of the lips or tongue, seek medical attention immediately!)
insomnia	• caffeine • overeating • spicy, fatty, or acidic foods that cause indigestion • going to bed hungry	• a small, bland snack, such as toast, cereal, warm milk, or yogurt, before going to bed
tooth stains	• coffee, tea, grape juice, blueberries, red wine, and other deeply colored foods and drinks	• drinking staining foods through a straw • regular brushing with a mildly abrasive or whitening toothpaste

SYMPTOM	CAN BE CAUSED BY	CAN BE ALLEVIATED BY *(continued)*
urinary tract infection	*no food causes urinary tract infections, but the discomfort can be exacerbated by tea, coffee, citrus juices, acidic foods, and spicy foods*	• *cranberry juice, at least 8 oz. a day* • *blueberries* • *water, more than your usual 8 to 10 glasses a day*
yeast infection	• *excessive consumption of sugar*	• *yogurt, 1 cup a day with active Lactobacillus acidophilus bacterium cultures (read the label)*

SEVEN DEAD-END DETOURS FROM HEALTHY EATING

Does the mere thought of losing weight or changing your diet leave you feeling hopeless, beaten down, a failure? Do you drag yourself to the starting line of each new race toward self-improvement already resigned to the fact you'll never finish it? Amid all the self-criticism ("I'm such a pig!") and rationalizations ("I could have stuck to my diet if only there were no holidays/vacations/stress in my life/food on the planet"), do you ever suspect that there's some mysterious secret to successful weight loss that's been eluding you (and about 100 million other Americans)?

If so, it's time to look neither to the calorie chart nor to the scale, but within. You cannot hope to achieve anything unless you understand why you want it. When asked why we want to lose weight, most of us respond with the obvious answers: better appearance, better health, or better endurance. But is that what we truly believe? Consciously or unconsciously, we look to dieting to solve a range of problems other than health problems. No matter what most of us may say, the driving force behind our diet resolutions is usually a hidden, unspoken desire for something else, something we are convinced will come with that smaller dress size, flatter stomach, and firmer thighs: a better love life, more nicely behaved children, a more attentive partner, or a less demanding boss, for example.

When we define success by these unrealistic and unrelated "goals," we undermine ourselves in two crucial ways. First, we diminish and fail to appreciate the real victories dieting does achieve, victories we can measure: the pounds and inches lost, the endurance that's improved, the pantry devoid of junk food. Second—and worst—every time a diet fails to improve other aspects of our lives, we throw up our hands, declare our diet—and ourselves—failures, and fall back into the old habits. Here's how to recognize and sidestep the seven dead-end traps that stand between you and the body you want and deserve.

1. New You, New Life?

What a wonderful world this would be if a smaller dress size came complete with a better life. When you put it like this, it sounds like the fantasy it is, yet many people burden each new weight-loss attempt with such doomed, unrealistic expectations. There are innumerable health benefits: lowered cholesterol levels (if you follow a lower-fat diet), lowered blood pressure, an increase in energy, newfound confidence, and maybe even a brighter outlook in general. Remember: Developing a new relationship with your body and with food can change how you look and how you feel, but not who you are.

. . .

Try looking at the other side of your fantasy, and remember that thin, fit people have problems too. Then toss it away.

2. The Unmotivating Motive

When it comes to struggling to achieve a healthy relationship with food, most of us have only two "gears": on a diet or off a diet. It seems that there's nothing in between. Too often, outside forces determine when and why we try to change how we eat. Whether in preparation for an upcoming event or in compensation for past sins, most of us diet for the wrong reasons, or at least for reasons that are never compelling enough to help us through the inevitable tough times. The trouble is, while these may appear to be good reasons to diet, they aren't strong internal motivators. They're enough to keep you breezing in and out of weight-loss programs because you feel guilty, bored, or stuffed into your jeans, but they don't achieve permanent results.

. . .

Find within yourself the real desire to change how you respond to food in your life and how you eat. Make change itself—not just the benefits that grow out of it—your goal.

3. *The Battle without a Plan*

Compare the times you've thought or said, "I have to lose weight," to the times you've outlined a precise plan for doing it. If you're like most people, you can't count the former because they don't make numbers that big, and you can't count the latter because it's never happened. And when I say having a plan, I don't mean just a list of menus and forbidden and permitted foods you got from a book or a meeting. I'm talking about the internal plan, the one that realistically and honestly takes into account who you are. What are your habits, tastes, schedule, and options? There's no point in vowing to never again touch a snack between meals if you have several young children at home. And there's no sense in defining your success by how long you can stay away from the foods you love.

Everyone needs a clear, well-thought-out, and realistic plan. That isn't always easy to do, because we're easily drawn to the most dramatic and drastic approaches. They're so different, we reason, they must work. But the fact is, they usually don't, simply because no one can stay on an unrealistic diet forever. There are many reasonable, workable diet strategies you can try: keeping a daily written record of your calories, eliminating all high-fat foods and replacing them with low-fat versions, joining a commercial weight-loss program, dieting with a buddy, or eliminating fats and meats for more vegetables and grains, to name a few. Ultimately, it doesn't really matter which you choose. The key is to decide on one plan, tailor it to your lifestyle, and then stick with it. That means don't switch to the latest fad regimen or start experimenting with diet pills or diuretics when the going gets tough.

. . .

Don't start a new diet until you can clearly and explicitly explain
what you will do to make it work most effectively.

4. *The Easy Road to Nowhere*

Theoretically, you might lose some weight by simply reducing your intake of calories and fat, at least in the beginning. But the real key to long-term weight loss and improved overall health is healthy eating habits combined with regular physical exercise. You'll lose weight faster and vastly improve your chances of keeping the weight off for good.

. . .

Remember: The easy way out leads you further from—not closer to—
your ultimate goal.

5. *The Quick Fix*

No one can accurately predict or control the rate at which the pounds melt away. That's why setting a deadline for achieving a desired weight often proves an exercise in futility. You can control what you eat and how much you exercise, however, and doing so not only will help you reach a desired goal but will set a pattern for maintaining your weight loss forever.

. . .

Remind yourself that your current physical state didn't develop overnight, and real change takes time. Honor your commitment to change your life as a positive act, not a chore.

6. *The Impossible, Inflexible, Unyielding Plan for Failure*

No matter how great your diet plan, if it's unrealistic and inflexible, it's doomed. Be honest. Do you really think you'll stand firm when faced with the temptations that come with dining out and attending celebrations? Do you really think Aunt Agnes will let you escape the Thanksgiving table without a slice of her pumpkin pie? Life is to be lived and enjoyed, and food's a big part of that. A diet plan that doesn't accommodate real life can't work. Beating up on yourself because "I blew it over the holidays/on vacation/with that chocolate mousse last night" is the dangerous first step toward abandoning your diet plan. Stop. Don't let these become excuses to quit, but rather reasons to continue your plan.

. . .

Learn to rebound. Expect—and enjoy—lapses and setbacks, then plan realistic ways to compensate through reducing calories or increasing your exercise over the next week.

7. *Failing to Identify Your Obstacles*

If humans were governed solely by logic, there wouldn't be diet and fitness books, magazines, infomercials, television programs, videotapes, and health gurus. A basic grasp of math, biology, and physics—not to mention common sense—would motivate us to eat properly and exercise. Often, however, other issues cloud our ability to "just do it." Obviously, food is more to us than just "body fuel," and many of us find our reasons not to exercise more compelling than either frightening health statistics or that sinking feeling when you admit you need the next bigger size.

Accept the fact that there may be illogical, emotionally based reasons why you relate to food and exercise the way you do now. Try to retrain yourself to think about these issues in a new light. Instead of telling yourself that you "don't know" why you polished off that box of cookies or that you "don't care" that you're too embarrassed to be seen in a swimsuit, admit how you really feel, if only to yourself. Consciously practice developing a healthy, motivating anger toward the situations that lead you to take comfort in cookies or keep you from finding the time to exercise. Stop hating yourself. You are not a "bad person," an "idiot," or a "lazy pig." Once you start thinking of yourself in those terms, you can't help but fail. You're simply someone who—like so many people—has learned some bad habits that need to be replaced with good ones, someone who's been a victim of decades of half-truths, pseudoscience, and hucksterism masquerading as "fitness advice." If you believe other, emotional issues are undermining your efforts, consider consulting a therapist.

· · ·

Learn to recognize and attack the real problems in your life,
not yourself.

STOP BEING TIRED

Fatigue is not only an extremely common complaint, it's the number one reason we often give for not being able to take care of ourselves as well as we'd like to. We tend to think of being tired as the natural consequence of leading busy lives and not getting enough sleep. And while most of us don't get either the amount or the quality of sleep we need (see "Have a Truly Good Night: Learn to Sleep," page 216), it accounts for only one form of fatigue. Individually or in combination, stress, diet, muscle tiredness, and hormones can make you feel worn out.

Here's a questionnaire to help you discover what may be making you feel so tired and what you can do about it. If three or more answers in any one category apply to you, correcting that form of fatigue should be your first priority. Note: If you feel chronically run down or if tiredness seems to have come on suddenly, see your physician for a checkup. Countless conditions, including many that are treatable, manifest themselves as a lack of energy.

IF YOU OFTEN FIND YOURSELF . . .	YOUR PROBLEM MAY BE . . .			
	DIET FATIGUE	HORMONE FATIGUE	MUSCLE FATIGUE	STRESS FATIGUE
dragging yourself out of bed in the morning	•			•
skipping breakfast	•			
sleeping past noon whenever you can		•		
experiencing muscle ache after you take a walk that's just a little longer than you're used to			•	
exercising less than you would like			•	
gaining weight even though you're conscientious about what you eat		•		
feeling listless by mid-afternoon	•			
ravenously hungry at dinnertime	•			
unable to sleep no matter how tired you are				•
not exercising at all			•	
napping so you can avoid an unpleasant task or situation				•
unable to focus by late morning	•			
noticing a lot of hair in your comb or brush		•		

	YOUR PROBLEM MAY BE . . . (continued)			
	DIET FATIGUE	HORMONE FATIGUE	MUSCLE FATIGUE	STRESS FATIGUE
rising from an afternoon nap feeling worse—namely, more depressed—and less energized				•
gasping for breath after climbing a flight of stairs			•	
thinking that you now feel more tired than you ever did before			•	
having skin that feels unusually dry		•		
feeling your heart race after moderate activity, such as vacuuming or walking quickly for a short distance			•	
having cold toes and fingers, no matter how warm your surroundings		•		
always feeling as if you're fighting a cold				•
having high-calorie, high-fat fast food for lunch	•			

How to Cope with Fatigue

First, don't be surprised if your answers fell under more than one category. Everything we do—or don't do—is interconnected. If you don't get enough rest or eat properly, you won't feel like exercising; if you don't exercise, you probably won't have an easy time getting the best sleep at night. That's the down side. The up side is, once you begin addressing the main source of your fatigue, chances are you'll begin to see a ripple effect in all areas of your life.

Diet Fatigue. Health and diet pioneer Adele Davis probably said it first, and it bears repeating because it's one piece of nutritional advice that never goes out of style: breakfast like a king, lunch like a prince, and dinner like a pauper. When you skimp on or skip breakfast, you start the day off at an energy deficit. Your body scrambles furiously to make it up by craving sweets, fats, and caffeine; holding back on energy you need to get through your day; and hoarding the fat you do have, so you don't lose weight. Throughout the day, eat balanced, nutritious foods with enough calories to power your lifestyle and maintain your fitness goals.

Hormone Fatigue. Your thyroid gland is basically the thermostat of your body, controlling when, how, and how quickly you burn energy. Hypothyroidism, while rare, often leaves people feeling unable to meet the challenges of the day. The good news is that hypothyroidism is easily diagnosed (through a blood test that is also part of any thorough annual physical) and treated through a temporary and safe course of hormone replacement (this is thyroid hormone, *not* estrogen, progesterone, or testosterone, the hormones usually referred to under the term).

Another form of hormone fatigue may arise during the transition through menopause. The symptoms of perimenopause and menopause that accompany declining estrogen levels often result in fatigue. You may want to consult your doctor about how you wish to manage these symptoms.

Muscle Fatigue. It's this simple: Muscles that are fit and strong can do more work with less effort than muscles that are not. Not only that, out-of-condition muscles are less efficient at extracting oxygen from the blood, forcing your heart—a crucial muscle that's been weakened by lack of exercise—to work harder. It's a vicious, potentially disabling and deadly cycle you can break easily with the addition of several sessions of moderate physical activity every week.

See "How Much Exercise Is Enough?," page 92.

Stress Fatigue. In and of itself, stress is not a bad thing (see "Managing Stress," page 223) unless it becomes chronic, long-term, and overwhelming. One major attribute of harmful stress is feeling that circumstances are beyond your control. Unfortunately, this describes many of the situations that prompt stress: having marital and family problems, caring for a sick child or other family member, dealing with pressures or uncertainty in your career. Women most often find themselves in a position in which they are forced to cope with one or, often, several such situations.

Since we often cannot change the situations that create chronic stress, we must focus on shoring up our physical and mental reserves to meet the challenges. Eat the best diet you can, with a special emphasis on vitamins B and C; eliminate other forms of fatigue from your life; give yourself a "stress vacation" every day, even if it's only for fifteen minutes and you never leave the house. Pursue a hobby, phone a friend, de-stress with yoga, meditation, massage, a good book, or a favorite television program.

WAKE UP TIRED EYES

Place a few metal tablespoons in the refrigerator until they're chilled—at least half an hour. Whenever you need to feel refreshed, lie down in a quiet spot, gently place the spoons over your closed eyes, and focus on something that makes you feel happy and relaxed. The rest will refresh you, and the cool spoons will reduce puffiness.

TAKE A REAL BREATHER

I've discussed adopting healthy eating habits and realistic exercise as ways to change your lifestyle. But there's a simple activity you can do to bring on positive feelings that will enhance all your other efforts along the road to well-being.

Breathing. We do it constantly and never give it a second thought. If we're still alive, we reason, we must be doing it right. Well, yes and no. We all breathe, but most of us don't do it as efficiently as we could, and few of us are aware that you can alter your mood simply by how you breathe. For centuries, students of hatha yoga have known what Western medicine is just beginning to discover: Much of how we feel depends on how we breathe. Here is a yogic breathing technique you can master in just a few minutes and practice anywhere, anytime.

Why does it work? Researchers have shown that any form of controlled, conscious breathing—whether the subjects breathe at a rate of fifteen, six, or three breaths a minute—substantially increases the level of oxygen in the blood. Heart patients in one study also performed better in tests that measured their response to exercise.

This breathing exercise is best done with your tongue in the yogic position: Touch the tip of your tongue to the back of your upper front teeth, then slide it up until it rests on the ridge of tissue between your teeth and the roof of your mouth. Keep your tongue there for the duration of the exercise.

The Relaxing Breath

The key to doing this exercise is pacing your breathing so that the relationship between the time you inhale, hold your breath, and exhale strictly adheres to the ratio 4:7:8, as outlined below. You want to be sure that it takes you twice as long to exhale as it does to inhale. The speed at which you're breathing isn't important. Don't hold your breath beyond what feels comfortable to you. Over time, you'll be able to hold it longer. For now, though, concentrate on maintaining those ratios.

Begin practicing this exercise at least twice a day. Right after waking, right before bedtime, and before meditating are all good times. Feel free to set other times, perhaps right after you get into the car, step out of the shower, or board the train for the commute home after a long day at the office.

1. Sit or lie comfortably with your back straight. Place your tongue in the yogic position. Exhale completely through the mouth, making an audible *whoosh* sound.

2. Close your mouth tightly. Quietly inhale through your nose to the count of 4.

3. Hold your breath for the count of 7.

4. Exhale audibly through your mouth to the count of 8. If you have difficulty exhaling with your tongue in the yogic position, try pursing your lips.

5. Repeat steps 2 through 4 three more times, for a total of four cycles. Breathe normally and observe how your body feels.

THE REAL WATER CURE

Water is without question the single most important ingredient for good health. We have on tap and free (or close to it) the miracle elixir of the ages, for all ages: the lifeblood of the earth itself, and the element we literally cannot live without. Maybe the fact that it's just about everywhere, colorless, tasteless, and free explains why we take water for granted. Or perhaps it's because few of us are aware of how much our bodies need and why. Read on and change the way you think—and drink—forever.

A 1998 survey discovered that while two of every three Americans knew they should be drinking eight 8-ounce glasses of water a day, half of them were not even drinking a third of what they need. (And, as you'll learn, eight glasses a day is the *minimum* you need to keep all your systems in peak condition.) As a result, most of us are walking around in a constant state of dehydration, further exacerbated by our consumption of supposed "thirst quenchers" that not only fail to add to our overall water intake but actually dehydrate us by ridding our tissues of water, along with crucial nutrients. These diuretic drinks include anything that contains alcohol (beer, wine, spirits, and wine coolers), caffeine (coffee, tea, cola, and other soft drinks), or phosphorus (in carbonated drinks, regular and diet, except club soda and seltzer). Water does everything from cushioning joints, regulating blood pressure and body temperature, and removing waste to helping move nutrients and oxygen into our cells, protecting our organs and tissues, and making the metabolism of food and body fat efficient. If you need a more dramatic reminder of where water should be on your list of priorities, remember this: You could live a few weeks without food (depending on how fat you are), but not more than two or three days without water.

How Much Water Do You Need?

The old eight-glasses-a-day rule is a good place to start. But when you consider that each day your body loses 6 cups to waste, 2 cups to sweat and evaporation (even if you don't feel as if you've been sweating), and another 2 to breathing, eight brings you up 2 cups short. And that's if you conscientiously drink the full eight, which most of us don't. You can make up a cup or two of water a day by eating juicy fruits, vegetables, and other water-rich foods, but don't depend on it. Also, surprisingly, you need just as much water in cold weather as in warm.

If you're overweight, you should drink an extra cup of water for every 25 pounds of additional weight. And you should always have on hand extra water if you will be out in hot weather, exercising, or anticipate being somewhere where water may not be readily available.

Most of us drink when we're thirsty, because we think that's our body's signal to "drink something." In fact, thirst is your body's way of screaming, "I'm dehydrated!" When you ignore your body's thirst signals over a period time, your body stops sending the signal until the condition becomes extreme. Don't wait until you're thirsty. Instead of quenching your thirst, you should think in terms of preventing it by proactively drinking water throughout the day.

The benefits of water are many:

- **WATER MAKES YOU LOOK BETTER.** It keeps your skin soft and plump (thereby reducing wrinkles and the sagging skin that often accompanies a dramatic loss in weight), your eyes clear, and your hair healthy.

- **WATER FLOATS YOUR MOODS.** Feeling cross, tired, exhausted? Got a headache? Drink a glass of water. Dehydration has a devastating effect on the brain (alcohol-induced brain dehydration is a leading factor in hangovers), resulting in an inability to focus, think clearly, and maintain an even keel emotionally.

- **WATER WASHES OUT FLUID RETENTION.** You read it right: Chronic water retention can result from not getting enough water. The explanation of this seeming paradox is actually quite simple. When you drink all your body needs, it uses the water for essential functions and then rids itself of the excess. However, when your body does not get all the water it needs, it goes into survival mode and "hoards" everything it gets, storing it in the spaces between cells just in case you never take another drink of water again. The result is swollen hands, legs, and feet. Taking diuretics only exacerbates the problem, since your body will hold on to the next drop of water, setting up a vicious cycle. How to break it? Drink enough every day. A sufficient water intake will also help flush out excess sodium, another culprit in water retention. Change your thinking. Remember: It's not the water you do drink that causes fluid retention, it's the water you don't.

- **WATER POWERS YOUR METABOLISM.** Your kidneys need sufficient water to clear the blood of waste products and toxins. When you fail to meet your kidneys' water requirements, they work at lower capacity and turn to the liver for help. Your liver's primary job is to metabolize glucose and stored fat, making it available to cells as energy, or marking it for elimination (that's how you lose weight). But the liver also clears unwanted and unneeded substances from the blood. When the liver pitches in to help the kidneys, it reduces the rate at which it metabolizes fat, and that slows weight loss.

- **WATER JUST MAKES YOU FEEL BETTER.** By preventing constipation, ensuring optimum muscle tone, and keeping your system clear of toxins and waste products, water makes it easier for you to feel your best.

WATER AND KIDNEY STONES

Those ten 8-ounce glasses of water a day can also help reduce your risk of developing kidney stones by 38 percent.

WATER AND OPTIMUM WEIGHT LOSS

Water is crucial to successful weight loss for several reasons. One is that we often misread a cue for thirst as a cue for hunger. Responding to hunger pangs with a tall glass of water will help you control your eating. Another is that getting all the water you need maximizes your metabolism. To "retrain" your body not to retain water and to signal thirst before you get dehydrated, try this: In the morning and at noon, drink a quart (4 cups) of water over a thirty-minute period. In the evening drink another quart between five and six o'clock. This will "shock" your body to restore a healthy water balance and make your efforts to lose weight and get fit more productive.

HAVE A CUP OF GREEN TEA

While water is absolutely essential, it's not the only beverage that can work wonders for you. Take green tea, for example. Though green tea is a relatively new addition to the American pantry, in China and Japan it has been considered a miraculous elixir of health for centuries. How can green tea improve your health?

Like other teas derived from the tea plant, green tea contains an array of components known to enhance health and well-being: vitamins C, E, and B complex, flavonoids, antioxidants, and fluoride, to name a few. Researchers have focused on the effects of green tea's primary component—catechins—for evidence that they can kill bacteria and viruses, reduce the incidence of cancer and other tumors, and help control blood pressure, blood sugar, and blood cholesterol. So far, the results have been promising.

Researchers at the American Health Foundation exposed mice to a cancer-causing agent, or carcinogen, found in cigarette smoke. One group of exposed mice was given green tea, the other was not. Forty-five percent fewer cases of lung cancer occurred among the mice who drank green tea. Another study found that green tea helped slow the rate of tumor growth in mice exposed to ultraviolet radiation, another known carcinogen.

But what does this tell us about green tea's potential effect on humans? In central Japan—where green tea is produced and the populace drinks ample quantities—the cancer rate is lower than anyplace else in the country. Researchers believe that the flavonoids in green (and black) tea account for lower rates of some cancers and heart disease among Asian men.

Green tea can be found in health food stores and on supermarket shelves. Several brands also include added vitamins and antioxidants. One word of warning, though: Green tea is not naturally caffeine-free. You can get decaffeinated green tea, which has the same antioxidant properties as regular green tea.

CAFFEINE CONTENT: HOW DOES GREEN TEA RANK?

BEVERAGE	SERVING	CAFFEINE, MG.
espresso coffee	2 oz.	120
regular brewed coffee	6 oz.	103
Mountain Dew (regular and diet)	12 oz.	55
Coca-Cola Classic (regular and diet)	12 oz.	47
Pepsi (regular and diet)	12 oz.	37
oolong tea	6 oz.	36
green tea	6 oz.	32
instant coffee, decaffeinated	6 oz.	2

Getting the Most Out of Green Tea

Use bagged tea instead of loose tea leaves, since exposure to air reduces available antioxidants. Don't brew the tea for longer than five minutes; it leaves the tea bitter and doesn't increase the level of antioxidants. Drink or discard the brewed tea within forty-eight hours, since after that it loses its antioxidant content. In the interest of food safety more than anything else, you should always store brewed tea in the refrigerator and discard it after forty-eight hours. If you can't cultivate a taste for green tea, stick with black. Black tea also contains antioxidants. However, green tea has an edge: catechins.

Getting Smart 2.

. . . .

Ann was in her late thirties, newly divorced, and miserable. Due to the turmoil in her personal life, she lost her high-paying public-relations job and, feeling lost, just began to eat. Her downward spiral hit its nadir the day she found herself refusing a job interview because she could no longer squeeze into her expensive professional wardrobe. "I turned on the TV, sat down with a half-dozen glazed donuts, and put everything else out of my mind. I'd do something about it tomorrow."

But tomorrow came and went, as did next week and next month. Finally her sister talked to her and convinced her that she was destroying her life. Later Ann told me, "My sister was right when she said, 'You know, you're just sitting here waiting for something that's never going to happen. You're waiting for a miracle—to put your marriage back together, to place the job of your dreams right in your lap. You've got to get out there and do something! I was waiting for a miracle. I just didn't realize then that I had to make it happen."

Ann came to me and confessed that she needed a personal trainer, because without an obligation to report to someone, she knew she would quit. She'd also had her share of fad diets and brief forays into the world of exercise. "I feel like I've done all this before, but this time it has to stick. I've got to make it work for me. What do I need to know?" We got to work, with a program that emphasized fat-burning workouts and better nutrition. Within three months, Ann was a new person. She'll jokingly remark about the real miracle—"that I finally got up off my fat rear end"—but she knows there was nothing supernatural about it. Whatever Ann accomplished, she did because she took control of her life and decided to make these changes. She took the first step and refused to stop.

BEFORE YOU START

Exercise and diet programs often fail us because we unknowingly "design" them to fail. How do we do it? We convince ourselves that the values and goals of a given diet plan or exercise philosophy should be ours. We set goals that are unrealistic, promise ourselves to "make time" that we just don't have, pursue activities that are not appropriate or enjoyable, or drop out before we see results because of injury or setbacks. We allow our health values to be determined from outside, not from within. No matter what you do, as long as you're doing more than you did the day or the week before, you're making progress, and that's all that counts.

- **BE HONEST WITH YOURSELF.** Think back to your last (or last few) attempts at exercising or eating better. Ann saved herself a lot of wasted time and disappointment by honestly assessing the weak point of her previous attempts to shape up. Ask yourself: Where did I get derailed and why? What can I do this time to avoid that pitfall? Were my goals realistic?

- **GIVE YOURSELF THE GIFT OF PATIENCE.** You may feel there are fifty things you'd like to change or do differently, but the more you try to do at once, the less effective or lasting those changes will probably be. There are some experts who feel that major lifestyle changes should be dramatic, all-or-nothing enterprises. You know yourself: If you respond to that approach, try it. But for most people, slow and steady wins the race.

- **GIVE YOURSELF DIRECTION: PRIORITIZE.** If you could choose only one goal, what would it be? Losing 5 pounds? Eliminating meat from your diet? Being more nutritionally conscious? Protecting yourself against future osteoporosis or arthritis? Finding the exercise program that's right for you? Write it down. Then list what else you'd like to accomplish in order of importance.

- **GIVE YOURSELF TIME, IN THE SHORT TERM AND OVER THE LONG HAUL.** You probably won't be a new person in thirty days, but if you improve any aspect of your health, you'll at least feel better. Give yourself time each day to focus on your health and grant yourself reasonable periods to accomplish your goals. It's probably better not to tie them to a single make-or-break externally imposed "deadline," such as your high school reunion. Two weeks is a reasonable amount of time to lose 3 pounds; it's not a realistic time frame for developing the endurance to run a mile a day.

- **GIVE YOURSELF REWARDS ALONG THE WAY.** If giving up your nightly cookie fix strikes you as a hardship, find more rewarding ways to spend that time: an aromatherapy bubble bath, a long-distance call to an old friend, a foot massage or facial, or a $3 skim-milk latte.

- **GIVE YOURSELF PERMISSION TO "FAIL"—AND TO WIN.** Whatever your lifestyle now, it's the culmination of a lifetime of habits, attitudes, preferences, and experience. It's not going to change overnight. People who change their lives for the better—people who lose weight and keep it off, exercise their way to health, and improve their lives in every way—will tell you it's a gradual process you grow into. Expect—but don't fear—setbacks. Figure out how and why each one happened, make a quick plan to avoid that problem again, and move on.

TO REACH THE ATTAINABLE GOAL

Give yourself lots of reasons to reward your hard work: Set a series of modest, attainable goals instead of one big one. You're more likely to lose the weight and keep it off if you concentrate on losing 5 pounds at a time. This works because it's a reasonable, manageable goal, and one you can feel good about and celebrate once, twice, a dozen times until you reach your ultimate ideal weight. And there will be something to celebrate: Just a 10 percent reduction in excess weight translates into a significant reduction in health risks.

BEFORE YOU START AN EXERCISE PROGRAM: TWENTY-ONE QUESTIONS

Be sure to check with your physician if you can answer yes to any of the following questions:

1. Have you been physically inactive for the past six months or longer (i.e., not participated in workouts at least twice a week)?

2. Are you a man over the age of forty? A woman over the age of fifty?

3. Is your current weight 20 percent or more over the ideal?

4. Is your BMI (body mass index) 36 or higher? (See "Body Mass Index: An Important Number to Watch," page 34.)

5. Are you pregnant or a new mother?

6. Would you describe your lifestyle as "sedentary"?

7. Do you smoke cigarettes regularly?

8. Have you ever been diagnosed with a heart condition? Have you ever experienced a heart attack?

9. Have you ever experienced unexplained pain, shortness of breath, dizziness, or other unusual discomfort at any time?

10. Have you ever experienced rapid, slow, or irregular heartbeat?

11. Do you have wounds or cuts on your feet that heal slowly or not at all?

12. Have you ever inexplicably lost your balance or fallen?

13. Have you fallen more than twice in the past year, for any reason (even ones you can explain)?

14. Have you experienced an unexplained weight loss in the past six months?

15. Have you experienced an unexplained weight gain or tendency to retain water in the past six months?

16. Have you ever been told by a doctor to restrict or modify your physical activity?

17. Do you regularly take prescription or over-the-counter medications that may cause dizziness, drowsiness, or diminished coordination?

18. Do you have any chronic pain in your bones or joints or loss of movement or range of motion?

19. If you are a woman, have you had any condition (bulimia, anorexia, binge eating, cessation of menstrual periods, low calcium intake) that would put you at risk for osteoporosis?

20. Do you have a chronic or serious health condition, such as diabetes?

21. Within the past year, have you been treated for a serious injury or illness or undergone surgery or extensive therapy of any kind?

BODY FAT: WHAT YOUR SCALE CAN'T TELL YOU

If you regard the scale as the accurate, impartial arbiter of fitness progress, you're giving it too much credit. The scale can tell you how much your body weighs—and even that can be skewed by water retention, a recent big meal, or dehydration—but it can't tell you what that weight consists of. And it's the proportion of fat to lean muscle tissue that determines: (1) if you're carrying a healthy weight; or (2) if your diet and exercise programs are producing results.

For instance, two women who each weigh the same 130 pounds could have entirely different health-risk profiles. In fact, a third woman of the same height who weighed 5 pounds more might be in better condition with fewer health risks because her "extra weight" consists of muscle mass, not fat. Contrary to popular belief, muscle does not weigh more than fat. However, it is much denser, so a pound of muscle takes up less space on your body than a pound of fat. That's why a fit 130-pound woman may look smaller than a plumper woman of the same weight.

It's also important to remember that improving your overall health is not a matter of simply losing 1 or 2 pounds every single week until you've reached your goal. If you're exercising regularly over several months, it's possible to gain a pound in new, lean muscle weight for every several pounds of fat you lose. On those days when the new muscle tissue first "registers" on the scale, you may mistakenly assume you've hit a plateau or you're just not working hard enough. Relax. This is one weight gain you should welcome. Not only is it transforming your body, it's revving up your metabolism, since it takes more calories to support lean muscle tissue than to support fat.

Most of our weight is comprised of bone, muscle tissue, and fat. Obviously, we can't do much to change the weight of our organs or bones. But knowing what proportion of your body is fat and what proportion is muscle gives you a good indication of how physically fit you are right now. Having a clearer picture of your weight-related health risks will help you set realistic goals and better gauge your progress than you could using standard height-weight charts or even the BMI (body mass index).

HOW MUCH FAT IS HEALTHY?		
BODY-FAT DESCRIPTION	WOMEN	MEN
Lean	less than 15%	less than 8%
Optimally Healthy	15 to 22%	8 to 15%

HOW MUCH FAT IS HEALTHY? *(continued)*		
BODY-FAT DESCRIPTION	WOMEN	MEN
Slightly Fat	23 to 26%	16 to 20%
Fat	27 to 32%	21 to 24%
Obese	more than 32%	more than 24%

How to Get the Most Accurate Body-Fat Reading

If you haven't heard of body-fat reading before, you're not alone. As more physicians learn its importance, it may become as common as a blood-pressure reading. Before you choose a method, bear in mind that even the most accurate method of measuring body fat produces an estimate, not an exact reading. And some methods are more precise and sensitive than others. Here are the pros and cons of each:

- **SKINFOLD CALIPERS.** These are "pinchers" a technician uses to measure the skin and the fat beneath in several key locations (such as the middle thigh, hip, and triceps). Using a mathematical formula, the technician then calculates your body-fat percentage. This is the cheapest method, the most widely available (most health clubs offer it to members for free or at a nominal cost), and the second-most accurate when performed properly. It can be the least accurate if the technician is not experienced. Other factors that may affect your results: having very loose skin or very firm skin; having a fat-distribution pattern that is uneven; or being measured soon after a workout or on a humid day (when your skin might be swollen from the heat).

- **BIOELECTRICAL IMPEDANCE.** This method uses a weak electrical current, which passes safely through your body from electrodes placed on your ankle and hand, to measure the water in your body. The results are then figured into a mathematical formula that gives the body-fat percentage. Generally speaking, the more water a body contains, the faster the signal travels. Muscle, which is about 70 percent water, conducts the current more efficiently than fat, which is 5 to 13 percent water. However, because this method is not directly measuring fat but water, you should know that being dehydrated, having just eaten, or retaining water (due to PMS or other health conditions) can throw off the accuracy of the reading. Avoid having alcohol or caffeine within twenty-four hours of your test;

don't exercise or eat within three hours beforehand. This test is available at health clubs and hospitals; it costs around $50.

- **INFRARED TESTING.** This method uses a fiber-optic probe that shines a beam of infrared light on the biceps. Fat absorbs light differently from muscle or other tissue, and these differences are measured, then calculated to produce the body-fat percentage. Infrared testing is available at sports-medicine centers; some health clubs and personal trainers use them as well. The test costs about $25, is highly accurate, and can be done at any time without any restrictions on your eating or activity.

- **UNDERWATER WEIGHING.** This is the most accurate method, but it does require special equipment and may not be readily available (you're most likely to find it at sports-medicine clinics and research laboratories). This method measures displaced water and the weight of your body underwater to determine body fat. It's easy enough: All you do is exhale, hold your breath, and then submerge yourself for about five seconds in a specially equipped tank of body-temperature water. Unfortunately, it can take some people many tries before they're able to fully empty their lungs of air. People who suffer from claustrophobia may find this method intolerable. The test costs between $50 and $100.

IF I'M NOT JUMPING ON THE SCALE EVERY DAY, HOW DO I TRACK MY PROGRESS?

Body weight can fluctuate dramatically, which is why making a daily ritual of weighing yourself is a mistake. Once a week is enough. If you find yourself retaining or gaining weight from week to week, honestly assess what you've been eating and how you've been exercising. Otherwise, forget the scale and pay attention to how you look, how you feel, and how your clothes fit.

BODY MASS INDEX: AN IMPORTANT NUMBER TO WATCH

How much should you weigh? That's a question everyone from physicians to fashion magazine editors have been answering for years. The old height-weight charts we grew up with rarely had any basis in medical fact (most were drawn up by insurance companies), and our society's concepts of what is healthy and attractive have changed. (If you don't believe me, remember that Marilyn Monroe often wore a size 12 dress.) Anyone who's ever embarked on a diet with a target weight knows the frustration of always fighting the last 5 pounds (which perhaps you should be keeping anyway) or hearing a health professional declare that "as long as your cholesterol's down, a few extra pounds can't hurt."

We know that those extra pounds come with extra health risks. The question is, exactly how do those pounds translate into increased health risk? Where do you start to worry? Five pounds? Ten? Thirty? Finally, someone has the answer. In the summer of 1998, the National Institutes of Health issued new guidelines after numerous large, extensive studies showed a clear association between body mass index and health problems. As a result, the NIH changed its definition of "overweight" from a body mass of 27 to 25. By this definition, over 55 percent of Americans are overweight, and anyone with a body mass of 30 or above qualifies as "obese." But even people who are not obese increase their risk of coronary artery disease, heart attack, stroke, high blood pressure, osteoarthritis, non-insulin-dependent diabetes, sleep apnea, and certain cancers (among them endometrium and breast) any time the BMI exceeds 25.

The body mass index—the product of a mathematical formula involving height and weight—provides a more accurate basis for comparison than the old height-weight charts. That's because the BMI gives a clearer indication of how much of that weight may be body fat. I say "may be" because muscle is denser than fat. Remember: If you take two women of the same height and frame, the one who is physically fit may actually weigh more than the one who is not. It's also important to take into account waistline measurements, since the fat that collects there is considered especially dangerous. If your BMI ranges between 25 and 35 and your waist measures more than 35 inches (40 for a man), you are at increased risk for weight-related health problems.

Higher BMIs signal increased health risk. Researchers followed 115,000 American women who participated in the long-term Nurses' Health Study. In 1976, when the study began, all of the women were between the ages of thirty and fifty-five; none had detectable cardiovascular disease or cancer. Over the next sixteen years, tracking only women who had never smoked and whose weight had been stable, the researchers found:

• the lowest mortality rate among women whose BMIs were below 19;

• mortality among women with BMIs of 29 and greater was more than double that of their leanest counterparts.

HEALTH RISKS RELATED TO BMI	
BMI	**HEALTH RISK**
20 to 25	very low
26 to 30	low
31 to 35	moderate
36 to 40	high
41 and over	very high

How to Determine Your BMI

For most people, the following chart is specific enough. If you would like to calculate your BMI even more accurately, follow these steps. Suppose you're 5 feet 4½ inches tall and weigh 147.5 pounds.

1. Convert your weight in pounds into kilograms by multiplying by 0.45

$$
\begin{array}{r}
147.50 \\
\times \quad 0.45 \\
\hline
66.375
\end{array}
$$

2. Convert your height in inches—64.5—into meters by multiplying by .0254

$$
\begin{array}{r}
64.5 \\
\times \quad 0.0254 \\
\hline
1.6383
\end{array}
$$

3. Multiply your height in meters by itself (or square it)

$$
\begin{array}{r}
1.6383 \\
\times \quad 1.6383 \\
\hline
2.6840
\end{array}
$$

4. Divide your weight in kilograms by your height in meters squared

$$
\begin{array}{r}
66.375 \\
\div \quad 2.6840 \\
\hline
24.7299
\end{array}
$$

Your BMI   24.7299

THE BMI CHART

height (inches)	54	55	56	57	58	59	60	61	62	63	64	65	66	67	68	69	70	71	72
meters	1.37	1.40	1.42	1.45	1.47	1.50	1.52	1.55	1.57	1.60	1.63	1.65	1.68	1.70	1.73	1.75	1.78	1.80	1.83

pounds	kilograms	54	55	56	57	58	59	60	61	62	63	64	65	66	67	68	69	70	71	72
95	43.2	23.0	22.1	21.4	20.6	19.9	19.2	18.6	18.0	17.4	16.9	16.4	15.8	15.4	14.9	14.5	14.1	13.7	13.3	12.9
100	45.5	24.2	23.3	22.5	21.6	20.9	20.2	19.6	18.9	18.3	17.8	17.2	16.7	16.2	15.7	15.3	14.8	14.4	14.0	13.6
105	47.7	25.4	24.5	23.6	22.7	22.0	21.2	20.6	19.9	19.2	18.6	18.1	17.5	17.0	16.5	16.0	15.5	15.1	14.7	14.3
110	50.0	26.6	25.6	24.8	23.8	23.0	22.2	21.6	20.8	20.2	19.5	18.9	18.3	17.8	17.2	16.8	16.3	15.8	15.4	15.0
115	52.3	27.8	26.8	25.9	24.9	24.1	23.2	22.5	21.8	21.1	20.4	19.8	19.1	18.6	18.0	17.5	17.0	16.5	16.1	15.7
120	54.5	29.0	28.0	27.0	26.0	25.1	24.2	23.5	22.7	22.0	21.3	20.7	20.0	19.4	18.8	18.3	17.8	17.3	16.8	16.3
125	56.8	30.2	29.1	28.1	27.1	26.2	25.3	24.5	23.7	22.9	22.2	21.5	20.8	20.2	19.6	19.1	18.5	18.0	17.5	17.0
130	59.1	31.4	30.3	29.3	28.1	27.2	26.3	25.5	24.6	23.8	23.1	22.4	21.6	21.0	20.4	19.8	19.2	18.7	18.2	17.7
135	61.4	32.6	31.5	30.4	29.2	28.3	27.3	26.4	25.6	24.7	24.0	23.2	22.5	21.8	21.2	20.6	20.0	19.4	18.9	18.4
140	63.6	33.8	32.6	31.5	30.3	29.3	28.3	27.4	26.5	25.7	24.9	24.1	23.3	22.6	21.9	21.4	20.7	20.1	19.6	19.1
145	65.9	35.1	33.8	32.6	31.4	30.4	29.3	28.4	27.5	26.6	25.7	25.0	24.1	23.5	22.7	22.1	21.5	20.9	20.3	19.7
150	68.2	36.3	35.0	33.8	32.5	31.4	30.3	29.4	28.4	27.5	26.6	25.8	25.0	24.3	23.5	22.9	22.2	21.6	21.0	20.4
155	70.5	37.5	36.1	34.9	33.5	32.5	31.3	30.3	29.4	28.4	27.5	26.7	25.8	25.1	24.3	23.6	22.9	22.3	21.7	21.1
160	72.7	38.7	37.3	36.0	34.6	33.5	32.3	31.3	30.3	29.3	28.4	27.5	26.6	25.9	25.1	24.4	23.7	23.0	22.4	21.8
165	75.0	39.9	38.5	37.1	35.7	34.6	33.3	32.3	31.3	30.2	29.3	28.4	27.5	26.7	25.9	25.2	24.4	23.7	23.1	22.5

Note: Figures rounded off to nearest tenth.

THE BMI CHART (continued)

height inches		54	55	56	57	58	59	60	61	62	63	64	65	66	67	68	69	70	71	72
meters		1.37	1.40	1.42	1.45	1.47	1.50	1.52	1.55	1.57	1.60	1.63	1.65	1.68	1.70	1.73	1.75	1.78	1.80	1.83
pounds	kilograms																			
170	77.3	41.1	39.6	38.3	36.8	35.6	34.3	33.3	32.2	31.2	30.2	29.3	28.3	27.5	26.6	25.9	25.2	24.5	23.8	23.1
175	79.5	42.3	40.8	39.4	37.9	36.7	35.4	34.3	33.1	32.1	31.1	30.1	29.1	28.3	27.4	26.7	25.9	25.2	24.5	23.8
180	81.8	43.5	42.0	40.5	39.0	37.7	36.4	35.3	34.1	33.0	32.0	31.0	30.0	29.1	28.2	27.5	26.7	25.9	25.2	24.5
185	84.1	44.7	43.1	41.6	40.0	38.8	37.4	36.2	35.0	33.9	32.8	31.9	30.8	29.9	29.0	28.2	27.4	26.6	25.9	25.2
190	86.4	45.9	44.3	42.8	41.1	39.8	38.4	37.2	36.0	34.8	33.7	32.7	31.6	30.7	29.8	29.0	28.1	27.3	26.6	25.9
195	88.6	47.1	45.5	43.9	42.2	40.8	39.4	38.2	36.9	35.9	34.6	33.6	32.5	31.5	30.6	29.7	28.9	28.0	27.3	26.5
200	90.9	48.4	46.6	45.0	43.3	41.9	40.4	39.2	37.9	36.7	35.5	34.4	33.3	32.4	31.3	30.5	29.6	28.8	28.0	27.2
205	93.2	49.6	47.8	46.1	44.4	42.9	41.4	40.2	38.8	37.6	36.4	35.3	34.1	33.2	32.1	31.3	30.4	29.5	28.7	27.9
210	95.5	50.8	49.0	47.3	45.5	44.0	42.4	41.1	39.8	38.5	37.3	36.2	35.0	34.0	32.9	32.0	31.1	30.2	29.4	28.6
215	97.7	52.0	50.1	48.4	46.5	45.0	43.4	42.1	40.7	39.4	38.2	37.0	35.8	34.8	33.7	32.8	31.8	30.9	30.1	29.3
220	100.0	53.2	51.3	49.5	47.6	46.1	44.4	43.1	41.7	40.3	39.1	37.9	36.6	35.6	34.5	33.6	32.6	31.6	30.8	29.9
225	102.3	54.4	52.4	50.6	48.7	47.1	45.5	44.1	42.6	41.2	40.0	38.7	37.5	36.4	35.3	34.3	33.3	32.4	31.5	30.6
230	104.5	55.6	53.6	51.8	49.8	48.2	46.5	45.1	43.6	42.2	40.8	39.6	38.3	37.2	36.1	35.1	34.1	33.1	32.2	31.3
235	106.8	56.8	54.8	52.9	50.9	49.2	47.5	46.0	44.5	43.1	41.7	40.5	39.1	38.0	36.8	35.8	34.8	33.8	32.9	32.0
240	109.1	58.0	55.9	54.0	51.9	50.3	48.5	47.0	45.5	44.0	42.6	41.3	40.0	38.8	37.6	36.6	35.5	34.5	33.6	32.7
245	111.4	59.2	57.1	55.1	53.0	51.3	49.5	48.0	46.4	44.9	43.5	42.2	40.8	39.6	38.4	37.4	36.3	35.2	34.3	33.3
250	113.6	60.4	58.3	56.3	54.1	52.4	50.5	49.0	47.3	45.8	44.4	43.0	41.6	40.4	39.2	38.1	37.0	36.0	35.0	34.0

Note: Figures rounded off to nearest tenth.

WAIST-HIP RATIO: ANOTHER INDICATOR OF RISK

In addition to calculating your BMI, there's another simple way to determine if you might be at risk for certain diseases. There is a direct relationship between bigger waist-lines and increased risk of stroke and heart disease, the leading killers of women (that's right, it's not breast cancer).

How do you know if your measurements place you in the at-risk category? Simple: Measure your waist circumference and your hip circumference. Divide the waist measurement by the hip measurement. Or use this handy chart. If the result is greater than 0.8, you're at risk.

WAIST-HIP RATIO (WAIST ÷ HIP)

hips (in.)	26	27	28	29	30	31	32	33	34	35	36	37	38	39	40	41	42	43	44
waist (in.)																			
22	0.8	0.8	0.8	0.8	0.7	0.7	0.7	0.7	0.6	0.6	0.6	0.6	0.6	0.6	0.6	0.5	0.5	0.5	0.5
23	0.9	0.9	0.8	0.8	0.8	0.7	0.7	0.7	0.7	0.7	0.6	0.6	0.6	0.6	0.6	0.6	0.5	0.5	0.5
24	0.9	0.9	0.9	0.8	0.8	0.8	0.8	0.7	0.7	0.7	0.7	0.6	0.6	0.6	0.6	0.6	0.6	0.6	0.5
25	1	0.9	0.9	0.9	0.8	0.8	0.8	0.8	0.7	0.7	0.7	0.7	0.7	0.6	0.6	0.6	0.6	0.6	0.6
26	1	1	0.9	0.9	0.9	0.8	0.8	0.8	0.8	0.7	0.7	0.7	0.7	0.7	0.7	0.6	0.6	0.6	0.6
27	1	1	1	0.9	0.9	0.9	0.8	0.8	0.8	0.8	0.8	0.7	0.7	0.7	0.7	0.7	0.6	0.6	0.6
28	1.1	1	1	1	0.9	0.9	0.9	0.8	0.8	0.8	0.8	0.8	0.7	0.7	0.7	0.7	0.7	0.7	0.6
29	1.1	1.1	1	1	1	0.9	0.9	0.9	0.9	0.8	0.8	0.8	0.8	0.8	0.7	0.7	0.7	0.7	0.7
30	1.2	1.1	1.1	1	1	1	0.9	0.9	0.9	0.9	0.8	0.8	0.8	0.8	0.8	0.7	0.7	0.7	0.7
31	1.2	1.1	1.1	1.1	1	1	1	0.9	0.9	0.9	0.9	0.8	0.8	0.8	0.8	0.8	0.7	0.7	0.7
32	1.2	1.2	1.1	1.1	1.1	1	1	1	0.9	0.9	0.9	0.9	0.8	0.8	0.8	0.8	0.8	0.7	0.7
33	1.3	1.2	1.2	1.1	1.1	1.1	1	1	1	0.9	0.9	0.9	0.9	0.8	0.8	0.8	0.8	0.8	0.8
34	1.3	1.3	1.2	1.2	1.1	1.1	1.1	1	1	1	0.9	0.9	0.9	0.9	0.9	0.8	0.8	0.8	0.8
35	1.3	1.3	1.3	1.2	1.2	1.1	1.1	1.1	1	1	1	0.9	0.9	0.9	0.9	0.9	0.8	0.8	0.8

WAIST-HIP RATIO (WAIST ÷ HIP) (continued)

hips (in.)	26	27	28	29	30	31	32	33	34	35	36	37	38	39	40	41	42	43	44
waist (in.)																			
36		1.4	1.3	1.3	1.2	1.2	1.2	1.1	1.1	1.1	1	1	1	0.9	0.9	0.9	0.9	0.9	0.8	0.8
37		1.4	1.4	1.3	1.3	1.2	1.2	1.2	1.1	1.1	1.1	1	1	1	0.9	0.9	0.9	0.9	0.9	0.8
38		1.5	1.4	1.4	1.3	1.3	1.2	1.2	1.2	1.1	1.1	1.1	1	1	1	1	0.9	0.9	0.9	0.9
39		1.5	1.4	1.4	1.3	1.3	1.3	1.2	1.2	1.1	1.1	1.1	1.1	1	1	1	1	0.9	0.9	0.9
40		1.5	1.5	1.4	1.4	1.3	1.3	1.3	1.2	1.2	1.1	1.1	1.1	1.1	1	1	1	1	0.9	0.9

A bigger waistline is also a predictor of increased risk for non-insulin-dependent diabetes, the most common form. A Harvard medical study that reviewed the histories of 42,000 nurses from 1986 to 1994 used a 28-inch waistline as the basis for comparison, and calculated increased risk as follows:

WAIST MEASUREMENT	INCREASED RISK OF DIABETES AS COMPARED TO A WOMAN WITH A 28-INCH WAISTLINE
30 inches 31 inches	2.5 times higher
32 inches 33 inches	almost 4 times higher
34 inches 35 inches	approximately 4.5 times higher
36 inches 37 inches	approximately 5.5 times higher
38 inches and larger	at least 6 times higher

The enduring popularity of fad diets proves only one thing: People will do almost anything to lose weight. And they'll do it with a few variations over and over and over again. The fact is, diets don't work because diets don't work. The Nutrition Research Clinic at Baylor College tracked three groups of dieters over two years. One group dieted but didn't exercise, the second dieted and exercised, and the third didn't diet but did exercise. Who kept the weight off? The group that didn't diet but exercised.

They may have new names, new gurus, and ever more esoteric theories behind them, but most fad diets advocate one of a handful of familiar and timeworn approaches. Here's what they're about and why they don't work over the long term, and may even be hazardous to your health. When you consider one of these diets, remember:

- **DIET FADS AND BODY FASHION MAY BEND WITH TRENDS, BUT HUMAN BIOLOGY NEVER CHANGES.** You need protein, carbohydrates, and some fat every day. As research into the benefits of plant substances and trace minerals develops, it's clear that we need to obtain them every day from fresh fruits and vegetables (which are woefully underrepresented in some of the most popular high-protein plans).

- **YOU NEED A CERTAIN NUMBER OF CALORIES EVERY DAY, NO MATTER HOW OVERWEIGHT YOU ARE.** It's basic math. If you starve yourself by drastically undereating, you set yourself up to either stop losing weight or to binge your way back to your previous weight (or higher) once the diet ends.

- **LEARN THE JOY OF MOVEMENT: EXERCISE.** If there is a magic ingredient to sustained weight loss, it's exercise. People who exercise take it off faster and keep it off longer. Period. And yet, if you look at the most popular diets, they lack the complex carbohydrates and/or the calories you need to be able to function in your daily life and pursue an exercise regimen.

- **IF YOU FEEL HUNGRY ON YOUR DIET, YOU'RE NOT LOSING WEIGHT, YOU'RE BUILDING CRAVINGS.** You don't have to feel hungry to lose weight, and constant hunger is a sign that you're not getting enough calories to maintain health, function well, or burn body fat.

- **IT'S ALL ABOUT DEVELOPING A NEW RELATIONSHIP TO FOOD, ACTIVITY, AND YOUR BODY.** A new diet and exercise program should be a learning experience, an ongoing transition between your old relationship to your health and a new, more positive one. Think about this: How can a philosophy that makes "enemies" of certain foods, that teaches us to fear and mistrust our bodies, that discourages exercise, or leaves us so exhausted and physically stressed that we don't even feel good *be* good? It can't.

- **THINK FOR YOURSELF.** Don't be swayed by the fact that this year's diet book is topping the best-seller list. That doesn't tell you how healthy, sound, or effective the diet is—only how desperate millions of people are to find a quick fix. Of course, many people who try them do lose weight initially, but that's only because people tend to eat less when they eat conscientiously. You would get the same results if you wrote down everything you ate for several weeks or simply decided to "do it."

Diets to Avoid

". . . I have not failed. I've just found ten thousand ways that don't work."—Thomas Edison

"Magical" Food Diets. In the early 1960s, it was champagne with every meal; by the late 1970s, it was a pickle. The mid-1980s brought us a rice diet; the early 1990s, one based on pâté. There is no single food or food group that can help you lose weight.

Super-Low-Calorie, Starvation Diets. A perennial, since early in the century, these endure under different names simply because a drastic reduction in calories will result in quick weight loss—for a while. Eventually your body defends itself by slowing down your metabolism, fat breakdown, and the rate at which you lose weight.

High-Protein, Low-Fat Diets. Early in modern diet history, carbohydrates—a.k.a. "starches"—were vilified, and protein was elevated to the status of miracle food. Excessive proteins (and remember, the average person already consumes far more than she needs) resulted in food cravings and ketosis, a potentially fatal condition that occurs when the body breaks fat down more quickly than it can eliminate the by-products of fat metabolism. No matter what pseudoscience they come wrapped up in, high-protein diets are inherently dangerous.

High-Protein, High-Fat Diets have all the shortcomings and risks of high-protein diets, with the added danger of whopping levels of fat, including saturated fats. If it's unhealthy to overdose on protein and fat when you're *not* dieting, what is it about dieting that makes it good for you? It makes no sense. The Sugar Busters diet is simply a new, even less scientifically supported variation on this theme.

High-Protein, Low-Calorie Diets offer barely enough calories to sustain life: about 700. Typically, people on these diets feel irritable and generally unwell—results of the one-two punch of ketosis and starvation.

Questionable Science. The early 1980s brought us food-combining diets based on the idea that it isn't what you eat, but how your body digests proteins, fats, and carbohydrates. Eating the wrong combinations (for example, protein with carbohydrates) supposedly results in "incomplete digestion," the "real" cause of weight gain. If that were so, we would all be grossly obese from the moment we began eating solid food.

Super-Low-Fat Diets are distinguished from other diets in that they seek to eradicate a specific weight-related health problem: cardiovascular disease. For people who have heart disease or are at high risk for it, these regimens are probably worth pursuing. But the inflexible restrictions are not for—or even necessarily healthy for—everyone.

Liquid and Liquid-Protein Diets. Though these may be indicated for people who are grossly or morbidly obese, and then only under a doctor's supervision, diets you drink rarely produce sustained results. It's an unnatural way of eating that leaves most people feeling so deprived, they're primed to binge. Learning how not to eat is poor preparation for learning a new way to eat.

THE FIVE ESSENTIAL TRUTHS ABOUT FOOD AND WEIGHT LOSS

Any diet philosophy that opposes these basic, scientifically established principles is doomed to fail.

1. **ALL FOOD THAT CONTAINS CALORIES HAS THE POTENTIAL TO CAUSE YOU TO GAIN WEIGHT.** No form of food is "more fattening" or more likely to make you store body fat than any other.

2. **THERE IS NO SUCH THING AS A "GOOD" FOOD OR A "BAD" FOOD.** Some foods are more nutritious and better for you, obviously, but there are no bad foods, only unhealthy diets and lifestyles. Empowering individual foods with moral qualities undermines a healthy attitude toward eating.

3. **EXTREMELY LOW CALORIE DIETS RESULT NOT ONLY IN FAT LOSS BUT IN MUSCLE LOSS AS WELL.** The less muscle you have, the fewer calories your body needs, making it even easier to gain weight, no matter how little you eat.

4. **A DIET BASED ON INFLEXIBLE GUIDELINES AND RESTRICTIONS THAT YOU CANNOT REASONABLY CARRY ON ONCE THE DIET ENDS WILL NOT PRODUCE LASTING CHANGE.** The secret to maintaining a healthy weight is eating right every day.

5. **WILLPOWER—OR LACK OF IT—DOESN'T CAUSE DIETS TO FAIL.** Diets do.

ANOTHER REASON NOT TO CRASH-DIET

A British study that tested women on low-calorie diets found that they were losing more than they bargained for. Short-term memory, ability to focus, and reaction time all suffered.

DO YOU HAVE A "SLOW METABOLISM"?

You've probably heard it a hundred times, and you may have even said it yourself. It's the timeworn lament of the overweight with all its variations: "I just have a slow metabolism," or, "No matter how little I eat, I still gain weight." Bottom line: You believe you can't lose weight because your body doesn't burn enough calories. Is this possible?

Yes and no. Some people do suffer from glandular—namely, thyroid—conditions that may result in a slower-than-normal metabolism. But these are extremely rare conditions. If you suspect you may have a glandular problem, you should see your doctor or an endocrinologist immediately. Chances are, you'll discover that you don't. Most of us grossly underestimate how much we eat—by 20 to 40 percent or more—and overestimate how active we are.

A recent three-year study has shattered the myth of the slow metabolism. One hundred people were placed (one at time) in a calorimeter, an environmentally controlled 9-by-10-foot box, for twenty-four hours. There was a bed for sleeping, a carefully monitored exercise bicycle (which the participants rode for a specified, equal amount of time), and even room service, in the form of identical meals (delivered through a slot in the door). The calorimeter also measured and recorded each body's heat production, oxygen intake, and carbon dioxide output. From these measures, the scientists were able to calculate how much energy each person expended.

The results: People eating the same food, getting the same amount of exercise, and living in the same environment burned calories at approximately the same rate. Now, here comes the tricky part: In 1995 the *New England Journal of Medicine* reported that when people lose around 10 percent of their body weight, their metabolism does slow enough to burn 15 percent fewer calories than before. There's one sure way to speed up your metabolism: Exercise!

WHY IS YO-YO DIETING BAD FOR YOU?

There's a lot of anecdotal evidence that people caught in a perpetual cycle of losing and gaining lose weight more slowly because their metabolisms lock into a "starvation" mode, resulting in a slower breakdown of body fat. Two 1996 studies, however, discovered that yo-yo dieting did not affect the basic metabolic rate. However, yo-yo dieting has not been "redeemed." It's always a bad idea, and if you find yourself yo-yo-ing, it's because whatever made the diet work didn't survive the transition to real life.

Before you try again, think in terms of creating health for life. Not only are yo-yo diets ineffective, they may have a negative impact on future health. A 1991 report in the *New England Journal of Medicine* concerned more than three thousand women who were studied for more than thirty years in the famous Framingham Health Study. Those who maintained a steady weight through the years (even if they were overweight) had a lower death rate and less risk of heart disease and some forms of cancer than those who gained and lost weight repeatedly.

THREE MEALS? SIX MEALS? DOES YOUR BODY KNOW THE DIFFERENCE?

Again, a one-size-fits-all "philosophy" collapses under the weight of scientific fact. The truth is, for some people three squares with a few nutritious, well-chosen snacks work best. For others, spreading their daily food intake essentially evenly over the course of six mini meals makes more sense. How can you determine which might work best for you?

First—and most important—don't be swayed by junk arguments like these:

- **FALSE: EATING MORE FREQUENT SMALL MEALS HELPS YOUR BODY BURN MORE CALORIES.** If that were the case, we could all snack with impunity. Some laboratory animals showed a tendency to store less body fat when they ate mini-meal style, but the same effect has not been shown in humans.

- **FALSE: THE MORE FREQUENTLY YOU EAT, THE LESS HUNGRY YOU ARE, SO YOU EAT FEWER CALORIES OVER THE COURSE OF THE DAY.** That may be true for a minority of highly self-disciplined people, but not for most of us. Studies prove that the more often you eat, the more calories you consume. And it's calories that make up pounds.

- **FALSE: FREQUENT SMALL MEALS GIVE YOU MORE ENERGY.** This is true only if you're the type who feels sluggish after a big meal or who is sensitive to dips within the normal range of blood sugar. (We're not talking about true low blood sugar, or hypoglycemia here; see "Low Blood Sugar: Do You Have It?," page 201.)

- **FALSE: LARGE MEALS "FLOOD" YOUR BODY WITH CALORIES IT CANNOT INSTANTLY BURN, SO THEY ARE MORE LIKELY TO BE STORED AS FAT.** Our bodies are much more sophisticated than that. Unneeded glucose—the end product of most of what we eat—is temporarily stored in the liver so it can be released to meet the demand over many hours after you finish eating.

- **FALSE: THE CALORIES FROM FREQUENT SMALL MEALS GET BURNED OFF FASTER, BEFORE THEY HAVE TIME TO GET STORED AS FAT.** If you eat more calories than you burn—no matter how, when, or where—your body will store fat and you will gain weight. Period.

IF THIS STATEMENT APPLIES TO YOU . . . TRY	3 SQUARES	6 MINI MEALS
No matter how complete and nutritious my meals are, I feel hungry most of the time.		✓
My job keeps me away from my office and on the road, where it's next to impossible to keep or find good, nutritious food.	✓	
Right after lunch or dinner, I fall into a slump, no matter how "light" the meal.		✓
I have a hard time getting excited about healthy, nutritious food unless it's part of a meal I can sit down to and savor.	✓	
Every morning around ten and every afternoon around four, I feel myself mentally fading away and all I can think about is having a cup of coffee and a candy bar.		✓

IF THIS STATEMENT APPLIES TO YOU . . . TRY	3 SQUARES	6 MINI MEALS
With my hectic schedule, it seems that I do everything on the run. I never have time for a real breakfast or lunch, so I seem to be snacking all day.		✓
Ever since I started a serious weight-loss plan, all I can think about is how deprived I am. My regular meals seem so skimpy to me, but I know what will happen if I start snacking too much.		✓
In our home, meals are family time: leisurely and relaxed. I'd feel uncomfortable breaking that routine.	✓	
I've failed on every diet before because once I return to my normal eating habits, I don't know what to do. I know I need to learn how to eat the right way when I'm no longer dieting.	✓	

What's best is what works for you, and the only way to determine that is to try eating both ways for a few days and see how you feel.

SIXTEEN COMMON EXERCISE MYTHS—AND HOW THEY CAN HURT YOU

Exercise myths are the old wives' tales of our time, repeated endlessly (with trendy variations) and embraced by both so-called fitness experts and couch potatoes. And unless you know better, some of them even make sense. The problem is that not only are most exercise myths factually, scientifically wrong, they can encourage behavior that produces injury or discourages exercise altogether. Protect yourself—and your workout program: Don't fall for these lines.

MYTH	MISTAKE	FACT
Exercise increases your appetite and your need for calories.	*Telling yourself as you spoon into that pint of Ben & Jerry's, "It's okay. I can burn it off."*	*It's true that exercise burns calories, but if you take in more calories than you utilize, you will gain weight, no matter how much you exercise. (See "Are You Eating Enough to Lose Weight?," page 88.)*
Exercise will increase your appetite, so you'll eat more and won't lose weight anyway.	*Avoiding exercise in a misguided attempt to reduce your appetite.*	*Exercise makes your appetite more manageable, not larger. Inactivity slows you down and increases your cravings for high-fat, high-sugar, and high-calorie foods to give you a short-lived boost.*
Exercise can't be worth the time and effort unless you can do it religiously for at least one hour every single day.	*Thinking that just because you can't exercise this much, there's nothing to be gained from exercising at all.*	*Three times a week for around 20 minutes each time will burn off a significant number of calories. Of course, if you exercise longer, say, 45 minutes to an hour, you'll burn even more calories. (See "How to Burn That Fat: Know Your THR," page 99.)*
You can't achieve substantial weight loss without exercising vigorously.	*Either pushing yourself too hard or ignoring less strenuous forms of exercise because you think they won't really achieve anything.*	*Moderate exercise such as walking can be effective in helping you lose weight. (See "How Much Exercise Is Enough?," page 92 and "When Is a High-Intensity, Calorie-Burning Workout Right for You?," page 97.)*

MYTH	MISTAKE	FACT *(continued)*
The more you sweat, the faster you lose weight.	Inducing dehydration by overstressing your body, using sauna suits, ignoring thirst and other signals that you need to cool down. This can be extremely dangerous!	There is no benefit to excessive sweating. Sweating relieves your body of water, not weight. You lose weight by burning calories, not by "sweating them out." (See "Water and Optimum Weight Loss," page 25.)
No pain, no gain.	Exercising to the point of injury.	Pain is not an accurate indicator of anything but injury. If you experience pain, stop. Do not resume your workout until you're certain you're not hurt.
Exercise is exhausting, and I feel tired enough already.	Avoiding it, not pushing as hard as you could.	Exercise is invigorating and energizing.
Exercise will exacerbate my (name your health condition).	Avoiding exercise altogether.	Under the supervision of a doctor or an exercise therapist, most people with chronic health problems can do at least some exercise. Consult your physician. Under the right guidance, chronic health conditions (for example, heart conditions and arthritis, to name two) often improve with the right exercise.

MYTH	MISTAKE	FACT *(continued)*
Once you find an exercise routine you like, stick to it religiously.	*Doing the same thing over and over until it gets so boring you start slacking off.*	*There are as many ways to exercise as there are days in the week: through sports, with videos, in classes and gyms— even walking or running with a friend.*
Always exercise on an empty stomach.	*Depriving your body of the immediate energy it needs, so that midway through your workout, you crash and burn.*	*Your body needs energy to burn energy. Eat light about an hour before you go for it. Yogurt and rice cakes are a good choice. (See "Make Every Bite Count," page 71.)*
Your scale is your best friend when it comes to judging how fit you are.	*Allowing minor daily fluctuations in your weight to discourage you and underestimate your progress.*	*Weighing yourself once a week is often enough. (See "Body Fat: What Your Scale Can't Tell You," page 32.)*
Women who work out with weights will bulk up.	*Neglecting an important aspect of total physical fitness— strength and muscle endurance.*	*Because women lack the male hormone testosterone, it's practically impossible for them to bulk up. (See the chart on strength-training fact and fiction, page 53.)*
Muscle turns to fat if you stop exercising.	*Deciding not to exercise at all, since "extra" muscle eventually will turn to even more fat.*	*Muscle fibers are muscle fibers, and fat is fat. Nothing can change them. What happens when you stop exercising is that your muscles shrink.*

MYTH	MISTAKE	FACT *(continued)*
Wearing ankle weights when walking, jogging, or hiking will improve your cardiovascular fitness.	*Strapping on the ankle weights and risking injury.*	*There is no scientific evidence that ankle weights help increase endurance or improve your fitness level. In fact, you risk injury to your joints, your posture suffers, and the weights will slow you down.*
You can change your body type through exercise.	*Becoming discouraged because you don't reach your goal.*	*Your body type is determined by your genes. However, you can use exercise to achieve goals that are suitable for your body type. (See "Why Body Type Matters," page 102.)*
Spot reducing— vanquishing fat from a particular body area by exercising that area—works.	*Concentrating on a very limited exercise repertoire at the expense of a true all-around fat-reducing plan.*	*You can "spot tone" specific muscles, such as abdominals, for example. But there's no such thing as "spot reducing." That's because when you exercise, you burn fat from all over your body, not just the muscles doing the most work. Where fat comes from and in what order it gets metabolized is determined by your genes. (See "Why Body Type Matters," page 102.)*

THE TRUTH ABOUT STRENGTH TRAINING

Despite all the evidence that strength training is a crucial part of any well-rounded, effective exercise program, many women resist it. Nothing can firm and tone you better or more effectively. Yet no other exercise regimen is as maligned and misunderstood as this. Many of us have a hard time thinking of strength training as a feminine activity. Misinformation about how strength training works, coupled with visions of Ms. Universe winners with washboard abs and masculine-looking biceps, often keeps women away. Most women want to be stronger and better proportioned, but not at the expense of losing their feminine curves or their femininity. Take a few minutes to sort the fiction from the fact, then drop your resistance and pick up some weights! First, some strength-training truths:

- **STRENGTH TRAINING IS EFFECTIVE.** Just three half-hour strength-training sessions each week can make a dramatic difference in how you look and feel.

- **STRENGTH TRAINING IS UNIQUE.** No other form of exercise can build, tone, and strengthen certain muscles—particularly in the upper body—as well.

- **STRENGTH TRAINING MAKES YOUR BODY WORK MORE EFFICIENTLY.** When you build muscles, you increase the ratio of muscle to fat. We all know that muscles burn calories while they're working. But the real beauty of having more muscle tissue is that it requires more calories than fat to sustain itself. The calories you eat are expended—effortlessly—instead of being stored in the form of fat.

- **STRENGTH TRAINING INCREASES BONE DENSITY.** The stronger and denser your bones, the better your protection against osteoporosis.

- **STRENGTH TRAINING BUILDS AND ENHANCES THE FEMALE BODY.** Contrary to popular misconception, you will not "bulk up" or attain a "muscle man" physique by strength training. That's because intensive training alone can't do it. You would need the male hormone testosterone too.

STRENGTH-TRAINING FICTION	STRENGTH-TRAINING FACT
Strength training won't help you get thinner, since it burns relatively few calories and adds pounds of muscle.	*Strength training does burn calories at least as quickly as walking does. And once you lose fat and gain muscle, your body will continue to burn more calories even when you're "doing nothing." Finally, the goal of any exercise program shouldn't be thinness, but fitness and better health.*

STRENGTH-TRAINING FICTION	STRENGTH-TRAINING FACT
Strength training may be great for building muscle and strengthening bones, but it does nothing for the heart.	*Research has shown that strength training improves cardiovascular fitness in three ways: (1) It lowers blood pressure; (2) it reduces levels of LDL cholesterol (the type that clogs the arteries); and (3) by strengthening your muscles, it lowers the chances that you'll suffer a heart attack during an episode of sudden exertion, such as shoveling snow or pushing a stalled car.*
Strength training builds muscle, and too much muscle mass reduces flexibility.	*There is a risk of losing flexibility if you exercise with weights and don't stretch during and after your strength-training session.*
Strength training will leave my body looking bulky and unfeminine.	*Most women cannot build large muscles on the same scale men can. The reason: testosterone. You can firm your muscles without adding bulk by working out with lighter weights and more repetitions. Working with heavy weights and fewer reps tends to encourage muscle bulk.*

YOU'RE NOT TOO BUSY TO EXERCISE: NINE TIME-FINDING TIPS

We can't create time or borrow time (now, wouldn't that be great?). And despite the rah-rah encouragements of organization gurus, most of us have little flexibility when it comes to meeting the demands of family and career. Still, virtually every day bears a hidden treasure of extra moments you can find for yourself.

1. **PLAN YOUR DAY.** The night before or early in the day, write down what you must accomplish, then prioritize your other tasks. Include among your top priorities eating well, taking your supplements, and getting some exercise. If you can't find time for a full workout today, resolve to incorporate some exercise into your other activities. For example, take the kids to the beach or to the park instead of the mall; bike to your friend's house after dinner instead of taking the car; vacuum the house tonight instead of reading magazines.

2. **EXERCISE REGULARLY.** It's easier to find time for those things we do every day than it is for those we do rarely. The exercise habit is like any other: hard to break once it's firmly established. If you're new to exercising regularly, be prepared to make the extra effort to talk yourself into choosing exercise over other time-consuming activities. Have your arguments ready; even write them down, if you must. Be prepared to argue your case. Believe me, it will get easier.

3. **LEARN TO BE SELFISH.** A recent survey found that the number-one reason women gave for not exercising is not having any time left over after meeting their responsibilities to their careers, their spouses, their kids, and the house. Once you start thinking of exercise as something you're doing for you, rather than just another among many demands on your time, it will be easier to find time.

4. **FIND THAT "MISSING" HALF HOUR: DELEGATE.** The figures are in: Women do too much. Look around your office or your home, then make a list of daily tasks you perform that take up thirty minutes of your time. Next, think of who else could perform those tasks instead, and enlist them.

5. **PUT YOUR EXERCISE PROGRAM IN PERSPECTIVE.** Instead of thinking about how much time you don't have, think of how much time you're spending on activities that pull you away from exercise. You've got to make some choices. When it comes right down to it, what would you rather have: a kitchen floor you can see yourself in or a bathing suit you could bear to be seen in? A meticulous, color-coded client file or the energy to serve those clients in less time and with a better attitude?

6. **TURN OFF THE TUBE.** Television amuses us, informs us, and relaxes us, all in the privacy of our own home. Take away its ability to entertain, educate, or distract us, and television viewing can best be summed up as thirty hours a week of sitting, including several hours of sitting and eating. What's wrong with this

picture? Cut down your viewing by even half, and you've added more time to exercise than most people need in two weeks. If you do watch, try to do it while exercising (jumping on a small trampoline, or using a treadmill, cross-country ski machine, or rowing machine).

7. **UNHOOK YOURSELF FROM THE LINE.** The telephone line and the Internet line, that is. Studies have shown that on average, most of us waste at least an hour a day talking on the phone, especially when we're home alone or stuck at work. Get into the habit of watching the clock. Don't be afraid to say, "Thanks for calling, but I've got to run," or, "I'd love to chat, but now is a bad time for me. Can I call you back later?" Or even ignore the phone altogether. (I have one friend who never answers her telephone in the half hour before, after, or during dinner.) If you must talk for longer than several minutes, go cordless and walk around inside or outside as you talk. If your friend doesn't object, walk on your treadmill or pedal on your stationary bike while you talk. And train yourself to view the Internet less as the wonder of the age and more as an improved form of home entertainment that combines the worst antifitness aspects of television and telephones.

8. **ORGANIZE THE REST OF YOUR LIFE.** Start out by establishing a routine for just one day a week (for example, all housework and shopping take place on Friday) or a weekly routine for just one unavoidable chore (say, bill paying every Wednesday night). One woman I know cut her shopping and cooking time by simply declaring Monday night chicken night, Tuesday night takeout night, Wednesday night pasta night, and so on. If your major workout days will be Tuesday and Thursday, make one of those nights takeout night, and let the kids or your partner cook the other.

9. **GET YOUR FAVORITE PEOPLE IN ON THE ACT.** Instead of talking on the phone for half an hour with your girlfriend eight doors away, invite her to take a walk with you. Toss Junior in his stroller, put Sissy in her wagon, or slip the collar and leash on Fido, and you're good to go.

DO YOU NEED A PERSONAL TRAINER?

Whether a personal trainer is a luxury or a necessity depends on you, your exercise history, and your personal goals. You might consider hiring a personal trainer on a long- or short-term basis if any of the following statements describe you:

1. The last time I worked out was PE class in high school.

2. I have started and dropped out of several classes and/or exercise programs in the past few years.

3. I'd like to train for a particular goal, such as running next year's marathon.

4. I've recently suffered an injury or illness.

5. I feel self-conscious exercising around other people.

How to Choose a Personal Trainer

Proceed with caution: Chances are, your hairdresser is more closely regulated than a personal trainer. In fact, in most states, there's nothing to stop a totally unqualified person from presenting himself as a personal trainer. Ask for recommendations from friends who have used trainers, the management at your local health club or municipal fitness center, and your physician. When you interview potential trainers, be clear about what you hope to achieve (for example, lose weight, train for a marathon, get into the exercise habit, shape up postpartum). Don't be intimidated by high-pressure sales tactics. Be sure you have a reasonably good rapport with your trainer; it's not something you can "add on" to the relationship later on. Go with your gut instinct.

Minimum Requirements for a Trainer

1. A professional demeanor. A personal trainer should be able to give you in writing information about his experience, background, philosophy, schedule, fees, references, and policies on cancellation and missed sessions.

2. Proof of liability insurance.

3. Membership in and/or certification from at least one of several nationally recognized sports-related organizations: AFAA (Aerobics and Fitness Association of America), NASM (National Academy of Sports Medicine), NSCA (National Strength and Conditioning Association), ACE (American Council on Exercise), or ACSM (American College of Sports Medicine).

4. The ability to listen to you and to articulate a clear, precise plan that addresses your specific needs and goals. Be wary of anyone who tries to impose his views of what your goals should be.

5. Willingness to give you a free or discounted sample session before you commit.

6. Experience with your particular problems. For example, if you're beginning training following childbirth, surgery, or a major illness, or if you are extremely out of shape, overweight, or have a chronic health condition, your trainer should have experience working with people like you. If you fall into this category, you might seek recommendations from doctors, physical therapists, and other medical professionals.

How Much Does a Personal Trainer Cost?

Fees vary depending on where you live, where the sessions will take place (in a health club or in your home, for instance), how long the sessions last, what kind of workout you'll be doing, and your trainer's experience and reputation. One way to save is to share sessions with a friend. The trainer may charge more per session to train two clients, but you'll probably each save over what you'd pay for private, individual sessions. Fees will also vary, depending on how much demand there is for a particular trainer. You might find someone who charges $25 an hour, while a famous trainer with a celebrity clientele can demand over $200 an hour. Ask around to determine the average range for your area.

Once You've Hired a Personal Trainer

Keep your eyes open for signs you're in good hands. No matter what your personal goals or what type of program you're following, every personal trainer should:

1. Design a program that addresses your personal concerns and gives you a solid, overall workout that provides flexibility work, strength training, and aerobics. Over time, your trainer should be willing and able to help you tweak your program to reflect your progress.

2. Keep close tabs on your progress. Your trainer should reevaluate you regularly, at least a few times a year.

3. Observe all safety precautions in every situation. He should be able to instruct you on the proper use of machines, proper exercise technique, and alert you to possible physical problems. When you're lifting weights or performing certain activities, he should spot you.

4. Explain your plan, the individual exercises, and how your body works in language you can understand. If you hear too much jargon, ask for a translation.

5. Recognize your limitations and his. If, for example, you have chronic back problems, you should be wary of a trainer who doesn't request a note from your physician outlining your physical limitations.

6. Train you with an eye to the day you'll be able to train yourself. Unless you feel you'd rather work with a personal trainer indefinitely, let your trainer know and perhaps even agree on a future date when he will "retire."

50-PLUS GREAT EVERYDAY WAYS TO BURN THOSE CALORIES

You don't have to carry around a pocket calorie counter to sharpen your sense of how your body burns calories. The counts below generally apply to a person who weighs 150 pounds, and they are approximations. (If you weigh closer to 100 pounds, multiply the calorie counts below by 0.66. If you weigh closer to 200 pounds, multiply the calorie counts below by 1.3.) A person who is more physically fit will have a higher muscle-to-fat ratio, so she will burn calories more efficiently and more quickly. Conversely, a person who is generally sedentary or who has a higher fat-to-muscle ratio will burn them less efficiently and more slowly. Calorie expenditure rates are also determined by how much you weigh. Generally speaking, if you compare two people with exactly the same fitness level and muscle-to-fat ratio, the lighter person will burn fewer calories performing the same activity as the heavier person.

ACTIVITY	CALORIES BURNED/ 30 MINUTES	CALORIES BURNED/ 60 MINUTES	NOTES
aerobic exercise, high-impact	231	462	Warm up and cool down.
aerobic exercise, low-impact	126	252	Warm up and cool down.
playing badminton	153–171	306–342	Shoulders, arms, and upper back should be in good condition.
ballroom dancing	126	462	Hips, back, thighs, and calves should be in good condition.
barbecuing a meal	85	170	Try not to inhale too much smoke.
playing basketball	240–300	480–600	Warm up at least 5 minutes, doing the activity itself in a slow, relaxed manner; this maximizes coordination and minimizes the risk of injury.
playing beach volleyball	272	544	
bicycling, outdoors	273	546	Follow the rules of the road; make sure your seat is positioned correctly; watch your back—keep your upper body relaxed and your arms loose.
bicycling, stationary, 12 mph	133	266	Set seat height so that your leg is almost straight when the pedal is in its lowest position; don't lean far forward (this can cause back and neck pain); ride with foot straps for greater comfort, efficiency, and fewer cramps; make sure the bike is sturdy.

ACTIVITY	CALORIES BURNED/ 30 MINUTES	CALORIES BURNED/ 60 MINUTES	NOTES *(continued)*
jumping rope	375	750	*Surprisingly exhausting; shoulders and upper body should be in good condition; jump on a flexible surface (for example, a wood floor, not concrete); wear good cross-training shoes with plenty of shock-absorbing cushioning.*
mopping the floor	107	214	*Be aware of your back; stop every 15 minutes to stretch.*
mowing the lawn, power mower	155	310	
playing paddleball	240–300	480–600	*Shoulders, shoulder rotator cuff, back, hips, thighs, and calves should be in good condition.*
shooting pool	77	154	*Requires flexibility and coordination; bend at the knees when shooting.*
playing racquetball	315	630	*Shoulders, shoulder rotator cuff, back, hips, thighs, and calves should be in good condition.*
raking leaves	150	300	*Be aware of your back; stop every 15 minutes to stretch.*
rowing machine	208	416	*Watch your technique; if you use your legs and gluteals incorrectly, you can stress your back; don't allow your knees to straighten fully when you pull back; don't bounce over or lean all the way back at the end of the stroke; your upper body should be leaning back at a 45-degree angle.*

ACTIVITY	CALORIES BURNED/ 30 MINUTES	CALORIES BURNED/ 60 MINUTES	NOTES *(continued)*
running under a sprinkler	204	408	*Don't forget the sunscreen; water reflects sunlight.*
running, 5 mph	273	546	*Good running shoes are essential; keep your head lifted, eyes straight ahead, shoulders relaxed, chest open, abs pulled in, arms close to body; run against, not with your back to, traffic.*
running, 10 mph	640	1,280	
running on a treadmill	425	850	*Start slowly; don't rely on the handrails for balance; if you can't keep your balance without them, you're going too fast; hold on until you feel comfortable letting go; keep your eyes straight ahead; wear good walking or running shoes; warm up and cool down at a pace slower than the aerobic portion of the workout.*
shopping for groceries	107	214	*Don't hunch over the shopping cart; squat—don't bend—for the items on the lower shelves; bend your knees when you lift groceries in and out of the cart and your car.*
skating, inline	238	476	*Requires a lot of balance, coordination, and concentration; beginners should take lessons; it's hard to brake.*

ACTIVITY	CALORIES BURNED/ 30 MINUTES	CALORIES BURNED/ 60 MINUTES	NOTES *(continued)*
throwing a Frisbee	102	204	Requires strong shoulder muscles to prevent injury to the rotator cuff— the four small muscles beneath your shoulder; warm up with internal and external rotation exercises.
tubing on a river	51	102	Wear sunscreen; warm up; kick up and down from the hips, not the knees; this can be exhausting.
vacuuming	120–150	200–300	Be aware of your back; stop every 15 minutes to stretch.
playing volleyball	150–180	300–360	Warm up at least 10 minutes, by playing in a slow, relaxed manner; this maximizes coordination and minimizes the risk of injury.
walking a dog	85	170	Keep the dog on a leash; bring water for your dog so he can drink every half hour; keep him off hot pavement—it will burn his feet.
walking, 3 mph	133	266	Wear comfortable walking shoes and clothing; walk as quickly as you can comfortably; pay attention to your form: relax your shoulders, widen your chest, tuck your abs in, keep your head and chin up, and look straight ahead.
walking, 4 mph	171	342	
walking, 4½ mph	220	440	
walking, leisurely	144	288	
weeding the garden	125	250	Be aware of your back; stop every 15 minutes to stretch.

ACTIVITY	CALORIES BURNED/ 30 MINUTES	CALORIES BURNED/ 60 MINUTES	NOTES (continued)
playing squash	over 330	over 660	Requires leg and upper-bod leg lifts, toe raises, biceps c triceps extensions, and wri. are all good conditioning e:
stair climber	325	650	Proper form is extremely ir do not grip rails; fingertips rest lightly on the bar in fr or on side rails; stand upri slight forward lean at the l even, moderately deep step your entire foot on stair.
swimming laps	231–272	480–544	Zero impact, which means you've been injured, or are overweight, or have arthri
swinging on a swing	68	136	Don't hunch forward; sit u eyes forward, abs pulled ii
playing tag	182	374	Wear good running shoes; move laterally with care; when tagging; keep your (forward at all times.
playing tennis, doubles	143	286	Stretch before playing to l and avoid injuries; stretcl relax muscles and minimi
playing tennis, singles	200	400	

WHICH HOME-EXERCISE MACHINE?

If I can choose only one home-gym piece of equipment, which should I choose to burn the most calories? A study at the Medical College of Wisconsin compared how many calories thirteen people used on six different machines: treadmill, cross-country skier, stair climber, rowing machine, stationary bicycle, and a stationary bicycle with push-and-pull arm levers. Researchers also compared calories burned at three different levels of intensity. At the two hardest levels, subjects burned the most calories on the treadmill and the least on the bicycles.

ELEVEN CLASSIC CALORIE FAIRY TALES

A calorie is a measure of the amount of energy produced by the food we eat. Nothing more, nothing less. And yet diet and fitness lore is filled with fact-free ideas about what calories are, how they work, and what we can do to control, limit, and banish them. Don't undermine your efforts by believing these.

1. **CALORIES FROM CARBOHYDRATES DON'T "COUNT" AS MUCH AS CALORIES FROM FAT.** A calorie is one unit of energy. It's a measurement, just as an inch is a unit of length or a cup, of volume. One calorie is one calorie, no matter what it comes from. Saying one kind of calorie is somehow different from another is like saying an inch of Rapunzel's hair is longer than an inch of Jack's beanstalk. Think about it. It makes no sense. There is one measurement in which the food source does matter, however, and that's the gram. A gram of fat contains 9 calories, while a gram of carbohydrate or protein contains only 4. But even when we're measuring grams, it still all comes down to calories.

2. **THE MOST EFFECTIVE WAY TO QUICKLY LOSE WEIGHT IS TO DRASTICALLY REDUCE YOUR CALORIE INTAKE.** On a strictly "bookkeeping" basis, it seems to make sense. The fewer calories you consume, the more fat your body will metabolize, and—presto!—the pounds disappear, at least at first. But anyone who's done a crash diet knows the results are as fleeting as Cinderella's golden coach. Starving might work if our bodies were machines and not finely

developed organisms programmed for survival. Your body recognizes a sharp drop in calorie intake as a life-threatening crisis. Once you reduce your calorie intake by 25 percent or more, your body protects itself by slowing your metabolic rate (so you hold on to fat you might have burned on a more moderate eating plan) and by raising the volume and frequency of the hunger alarm. This metabolic slowdown also kicks in once you lose about 10 percent of your body weight.

3. **JUST CUT OUT MOST OF THE FAT AND YOU'LL NEVER HAVE TO DIET AGAIN.** This might be true if you replaced your dietary fat with naturally low-fat whole grains, fruits, vegetables, and skim milk and other low-fat dairy products. The "fat is all that matters" approach of the 1990s reflects a promising premise based on some solid, if limited, information. It stands to reason that if most people are eating too much fat, they will probably lose weight by eliminating fat. What the experts didn't account for—again—is the body's ability to find ways to get what it needs and wants however it can. Our bodies crave a certain amount of dietary fat. Studies have shown that people who eat extremely low fat or nonfat diets usually eat more carbohydrates, as if their bodies were trying to compensate for the "missing" fat. Plus, processed low-fat and fat-free foods often contain as many calories as the high-fat food they replace.

"FAT-FREE" AND "LOW-FAT" DON'T MEAN "LOW-CALORIE"

Most of us should restrict our daily fat intake to 25 percent to 30 percent of total calories, so lower-fat versions are sometimes a better choice. Just be aware that they don't come "free." "Fat-free" and "low-fat" are not synonymous with "low-calorie." As you can see from the chart below (and that on page 82), the difference in calories between high- and low-fat versions of the same food can be negligible. Not to advocate eating a high-fat diet, but if you are really craving the rich taste of real chocolate chip cookies, why not just eat two real cookies rather than four lower-fat versions? You'd save half the calories and consume less than a gram more fat than you would have eaten with four lower-fat cookies. Before you help yourself to the next "lower-fat" helping, compare the labels and see how much you're really saving—in both fat grams and calories.

cookie	calories	fat, gr.
vanilla wafer, 4 cookies, 6 grams each, lower-fat	104	3.6
vanilla wafer, 4 cookies, 6 grams each, higher-fat	112	4.6
chocolate chip, 4 cookies, 6 grams each, lower fat	180	6
chocolate chip, 4 cookies, 6 grams each, higher fat	192	12.8

4. **CALORIES FROM FAT OR CALORIES FROM PROTEIN DON'T COUNT IF YOU AVOID CARBOHYDRATES.** Is this because carbohydrates cast a wicked spell that makes fat and protein calories stick? This particular slice of junk science simply refuses to die. The fact is, if you follow one of these diets, you'll probably see results only because we take in most of our calories in carbohydrates. The only reason this works is because your body is responding to the restricted calories— not the restricted carbohydrates. (See "Don't Be Dazzled by Fad Diets," page 41.)

5. **FOODS SUCH AS CELERY AND GRAPEFRUIT HAVE "NEGATIVE CALORIES" BECAUSE YOU BURN LOTS OF FUEL DIGESTING THEM.** This is based on the idea that the body uses more calories to digest some foods than others. The truth is, the number of calories your body expends digesting your food remains basically consistent, no matter what you eat. There is no such thing as a "negative-calorie" food.

6. **OLIVE OIL IS HEALTHIER AND LESS FATTENING THAN OTHER OILS.** This is half-true. Because it is monounsaturated, olive oil is healthier than other oils. But as far as calories are concerned, olive oil weighs in with the same 125 calories per tablespoon as all the rest.

7. **IF YOUR DIET IS EXTREMELY HEALTHY (I.E., VEGETARIAN, ORGANIC, EXTREMELY LOW FAT), YOU CAN EAT WHATEVER YOU WANT. THE CALORIES WILL "TAKE CARE OF THEMSELVES."** We can't seem to escape the mind trap of thinking that if something is good for us, more of it must be better. Calories from vegetarian, organic, or low-fat foods still count. However, people who eat diets full of whole grains, fresh fruits, and vegetables—in other words, real food— often find they are more satisfied and less likely to overeat than those who live on heavily processed foods.

8. **THE BODY HAS ITS OWN WISDOM. YOU'RE ONLY HUNGRY WHEN YOUR BODY NEEDS FOOD; OVEREATING ONE DAY WILL BE OFFSET BY BEING LESS HUNGRY THE NEXT.** If only! Our bodies do know what we need, but most of us stopped listening years ago. Now most of us don't know to drink water until we become dehydrated, or when to stop eating. True physiological hunger is but one reason we feel like eating. Stress, depression, a need for comfort, loneliness, and certain social situations and activities can all send out the hunger signal. It's no wonder that many people don't even know what "normal" hunger feels like anymore. If you "trust" your body to manage your food intake, you'll be sorry.

9. **THERE ARE POWERFUL FOODS AND FOOD SUPPLEMENTS THAT "BURN," "MELT," AND "EAT AWAY" CALORIES.** If that were true, we'd all be popping these magic substances with every meal. Alas, nothing can neutralize a calorie except burning it metabolically.

10. **"COUNTING CALORIES" DOESN'T WORK.** True, there's more to achieving long-term weight loss and weight management than just counting calories. You have to eat the right foods and exercise too. But not having even the vaguest idea of what foods or types of foods are calorie-dense and which are not is asking for trouble. The calorie is really the only means we have of determining what we're taking in and what we're burning.

11. **ALL I NEED TO KNOW ABOUT CALORIES I CAN READ OFF THE PACKAGE LABEL.** The Nutrition Facts labels that now appear on all prepared and packaged foods do take the guesswork out of healthy eating. The problem is that most of us focus on the calorie count given for a single serving, then help ourselves to the equivalent of one and half, two, even three or more servings without adding in the difference. On average, overweight people underestimate their daily caloric intake by about 40 percent. And people who maintain a healthy weight usually underestimate theirs by 20 percent. Wake up! Learn to recognize what a portion really looks like, even if you have to measure each serving. If you find it difficult to control yourself when it comes to desserts and treats, try buying single-serving packs: sorbet and ice cream in pops instead of in pints; puddings and gelatins in "snack packs" instead of tubs; chips in lunchbox-size mini bags instead of jumbo 2-pound packs; soda in single-serving 12-ounce cans or bottles, not liters or Big Gulps.

MAKE EVERY BITE COUNT

For too long the words *diet* and *healthy eating* have been synonymous with deprivation. But eating better does not mean starving yourself. In fact, you have to fuel up to trim down. Here's how.

- **PLAN FOR SNACK ATTACKS.** Keep healthful munchies within easy reach. Fruits and vegetables make the best snacks because they're loaded with nutrients and are low in calories. Good bets: baby carrots, celery, apples, grapes, pretzels, plain popcorn, string cheese, hot peppers, salsa, soy chips, and unsalted roasted soybeans.

- **FACE IT: SIZE MATTERS.** Learn to identify what constitutes the proper portion size—it's a lot smaller than you think. A 3-ounce serving of meat, for example, is about the width and height of a deck of playing cards. When you eat out, be aware that most restaurants customarily serve portions that are twice, even three times a normal portion. Ask for the doggie bag.

- **BE A WATER BABY.** To keep your body hydrated, especially when you're working out, you should drink at least eight 8-ounce glasses of water every day— including before, during, and after your workout. Sometimes we feel hungry when we're actually dehydrated. Before you snack, drink a tall glass of water and then see how you feel. (See "The Real Water Cure," page 22.)

- **HAVE BREAKFAST.** Some studies suggest that people who skip breakfast are more likely to either overeat or snack later in the day. If you wake up not feeling hungry, it may mean you're eating too much too late, keeping your blood sugar high overnight. Try eating a smaller dinner and no after-dinner snacks and see if your breakfast appetite returns. Best bets for breakfast: hot or cold cereals, because they contain vitamins, minerals, complex carbohydrates, and fiber. (See "Join the Breakfast Club," page 199.)

- **SAY BYE-BYE, ALCOHOL.** While a glass of red wine now and then is fine, and probably even good for you, alcohol offers empty calories and can lead to impulsive eating later on.

- **GET SOME SATISFACTION.** At mealtime, make every bite count by choosing foods that are nutritious, filling, and enjoyable to you. Certain foods—such as baked potatoes, oatmeal, and pasta—are more satisfying than others, making it easier to stave off that between-meal hunger.

- **LEARN TO LOVE FOOD FOR QUALITIES OTHER THAN TASTE.** About half of the sensual pleasure we derive from food comes from its scent. Learning to eat more conscientiously—to appreciate and savor how food looks, feels, smells, and tastes—will make the experience of eating more satisfying. Instead of focusing on how that apple is not like the eclair you really wanted, consider its size, shape, color, texture, scent, and the fact that it grew from a tree, not a factory.

- **GET MILK.** Make sure you're getting enough calcium (at least 1,000 mg. a day) through milk, cheese, yogurt, or supplements. (See "Learn the B, C, D's of Better Bones," page 186.)

- **SNACKING ON THE GO.** If you've been sticking to your diet plan but find you're hungry before your workout, here are a few things you can grab—along with two glasses of water—up to thirty minutes before you exercise: one banana; half a plain bagel; 1/2 cup dried fruit; rice cakes; air-popped popcorn (delicious sprinkled with low-fat Parmesan cheese); or fat-free pretzels.

- **GIVE IT A REST.** If you've finished your meal and still feel hungry, wait twenty minutes before reaching for seconds. That is the amount of time it takes for your brain to process the signal that you're no longer hungry. When you think about how many calories you can consume in twenty minutes—calories you don't need—it's easy to see where the extra pounds come from.

- **THINK—AND EAT—SMALL.** If you want to lose weight and keep your energy level up, eat small meals throughout the day. And don't reason that eating nothing is better than eating small. When you skip a meal, your energy flags, and you're more likely to grab for the sweet pick-me-up or to overeat at your next meal.

KNOW YOUR FOOD

Now that most food labels include "Nutrition Facts," you might assume they tell you all you need to know. Beyond serving sizes, calories, fat calories, total fat, saturated fat, cholesterol, sodium, carbohydrates, fiber, sugars, protein, vitamins, calcium, and iron, what else could there be *to* know? Actually, a lot.

Every calorie you eat comes from one of three types of food: protein, fat, or carbohydrate. One essential key to healthy eating is making sure you consume all three every day in the correct proportions.

Carbohydrates	at least 55 percent
Protein	no more than 20 percent
Fat	20 to 30 percent

While the Nutrition Facts tell us the number and type of fat grams in a serving, they do not provide information on what percentage of the food fat constitutes. (And don't be confused by the percentage column that reads "%DV." That refers to the percentage of the Daily Values based on a 2,000-calorie diet, not the percentage of fat in the food.) So how do you determine how a food's fat grams translate into daily fat-calorie percentages? Here's a quick, easy-to-remember formula:

1. Look for the number of fat grams under Nutrition Facts and multiply that number by 30 (or whatever percentage you wish to keep your fat consumption at or under).

2. Look for the total number of calories under Nutrition Facts.

3. Find the difference between the two. That number will be the food's fat-calorie percentage, and shouldn't exceed the percentage you've chosen as your desired daily fat consumption.

Here's how it works. If you're considering eating a muffin that contains 7 grams of fat and 150 calories, your calculation would look like this:

$$\begin{array}{rl} 7 & \text{grams of fat} \\ \times\ 30 & \text{desired percentage of daily fat intake} \\ \hline 210 & \end{array}$$

Because the muffin contains 150 total calories, and the formula sum is 210, the difference between the two is 60 (210 − 150 = 60). You know, then, that its fat content exceeds 30 percent.

Now, let's say the same 150-calorie muffin contained 4 grams of fat.

$$
\begin{array}{rl}
4 & \text{grams of fat} \\
\times\ 30 & \text{desired percentage of daily fat intake} \\
\hline
120 &
\end{array}
$$

Since 120 is less than 150, this muffin falls within the 30 percent range.

Or, let's assume you're aiming to reduce your fat intake to 25 percent of your daily calories. Would the 150-calorie, lower-fat muffin make the grade?

$$
\begin{array}{rl}
4 & \text{grams of fat} \\
\times\ 25 & \text{desired percentage of daily fat intake} \\
\hline
100 &
\end{array}
$$

Yes, because 100 is less than 150.

You can also refer to the following charts: One is for 25 percent and the other for 30 percent daily fat intake. Find the number of fat grams in the left-hand column and the number of calories per serving at the top. If the number that appears where they meet is a negative number or a 0, the fat content is at or below the recommended daily fat intake.

Does this mean you should never eat any food that gets more than 30 percent of its calories from fat? No. Just use common sense. If you must splurge on a serving of fettuccine Alfredo or Ben & Jerry's Chocolate Chip Cookie Dough Ice Cream, make sure the rest of the day's calories come from low- or no-fat choices.

25 PERCENT DAILY FAT INTAKE

calories fat gr.	100	150	200	250	300	350	400	450	500
1	−75	−125	−175	−225	−275	−325	−375	−425	−475
2	−50	−100	−150	−200	−250	−300	−350	−400	−450
3	−25	−75	−125	−175	−225	−275	−325	−375	−425
4	0	−50	−100	−150	−200	−250	−300	−350	−400
5	25	−25	−75	−125	−175	−225	−275	−325	−375
6	50	0	−50	−100	−150	−200	−250	−300	−350
7	75	25	−25	−75	−125	−175	−225	−275	−325
8	100	50	0	−50	−100	−150	−200	−250	−300
9	125	75	25	−25	−75	−125	−175	−225	−275
10	150	100	50	0	−50	−100	−150	−200	−250

25 PERCENT DAILY FAT INTAKE (continued)

calories fat gr.	100	150	200	250	300	350	400	450	500
11	175	125	75	25	−25	−75	−125	−175	−225
12	200	150	100	50	0	−50	−100	−150	−200
13	225	175	125	75	25	−25	−75	−125	−175
14	250	200	150	100	50	0	−50	−100	−150
15	275	225	175	125	75	25	−25	−75	−125
16	300	250	200	150	100	50	0	−50	−100
17	325	275	225	175	125	75	25	−25	−75
18	350	300	250	200	150	100	50	0	−50
19	375	325	275	225	175	125	75	25	−25
20	400	350	300	250	200	150	100	50	0
21	425	375	325	275	225	175	125	75	25
22	450	400	350	300	250	200	150	100	50
23	475	425	375	325	275	225	175	125	75
24	500	450	400	350	300	250	200	150	100
25	525	475	425	375	325	275	225	175	125
26	550	500	450	400	350	300	250	200	150
27	575	525	475	425	375	325	275	225	175
28	600	550	500	450	400	350	300	250	200
29	625	575	525	475	425	375	325	275	225
30	650	600	550	500	450	400	350	300	250

30 PERCENT DAILY FAT INTAKE

calories fat gr.	100	150	200	250	300	350	400	450	500
1	−70	−120	−170	−220	−270	−320	−370	−420	−470
2	−40	−90	−140	−190	−240	−290	−340	−390	−440
3	−10	−60	−110	−160	−210	−260	−310	−360	−410
4	20	−30	−80	−130	−180	−230	−280	−330	−380
5	50	0	−50	−100	−150	−200	−250	−300	−350
6	80	30	−20	−70	−120	−170	−220	−270	−320
7	110	60	10	−40	−90	−140	−190	−240	−290
8	140	90	40	−10	−60	−110	−160	−210	−260
9	170	120	70	20	−30	−80	−130	−180	−230
10	200	150	100	50	0	−50	−100	−150	−200
11	230	180	130	80	30	−20	−70	−120	−170

30 PERCENT DAILY FAT INTAKE *(continued)*

calories fat gr.	100	150	200	250	300	350	400	450	500
12	260	210	160	110	60	10	–40	–90	–140
13	290	240	190	140	90	40	–10	–60	–110
14	320	270	220	170	120	70	20	–30	–80
15	350	300	250	200	150	100	50	0	–50
16	380	330	280	230	180	130	80	30	–20
17	410	360	310	260	210	160	110	60	10
18	440	390	340	290	240	190	140	90	40
19	470	420	370	320	270	220	170	120	70
20	500	450	400	350	300	250	200	150	100
21	530	480	430	380	330	280	230	180	130
22	560	510	460	410	360	310	260	210	160
23	590	540	490	440	390	340	290	240	190
24	620	570	520	470	420	370	320	270	220
25	650	600	550	500	450	400	350	300	250
26	680	630	580	530	480	430	380	330	280
27	710	660	610	560	510	460	410	360	310
28	740	690	640	590	540	490	440	390	340
29	770	720	670	620	570	520	470	420	370
30	800	750	700	650	600	550	500	450	400

REMEMBER: SUGAR IS SUGAR IS SUGAR

Chemically speaking, sugar is a simple carbohydrate, a quick-acting fuel for the body. Nothing more, nothing less. Our relationship to sugar is complicated, because it's the sweet treat we crave but that we rarely indulge without giving at least a passing thought to its real and purported evils, from tooth decay to cancer. Fear of sugar and its attendant calories have sweetened the pot for artificial sweeteners, which have a troubled history of their own. (See "Is Your Diet Soda Undoing Your Diet?," page 82.)

We often speak of sugar's calories as being "empty," because all sugar offers is pure energy without any nutritional benefit. But our bodies need energy. The problem with sugar is that we consume far too much of it. White granulated "table" sugar, brown sugar, honey, fructose, glucose—to your body, it's all the same. No form of sugar has a nutritional advantage over any other, with the exception of molasses, which contains iron. In fact, honey and brown, or "natural," sugar have more calories per teaspoon than white sugar. And while we may have a very strong desire for sugar, there is no scientific evidence that sugar is truly addictive in the same sense that caffeine is.

What is addictive are the bad eating habits that prompt intense sugar cravings. And there's no question about it: We are a nation with a sweet tooth, with a per-capita consumption of 150 pounds of sugar in its many forms every year. How much sugar is too much? First, there is no minimum requirement for sugar. You could live without it, but it doesn't seem that many of us do. In 1994, the average daily intake was 45 teaspoons: That's nearly 300 percent over what the U.S. Department of Agriculture suggests for someone on a 2,000-calorie diet. The recommended maximum 12 teaspoons (or 1/4 cup) a day may sound like a lot of sugar, but it's really not, especially since so much of the sugar we consume is "invisible"—included in such prepared products as breads, ketchup, salad dressings, soups, frozen vegetables with special sauces, and other sauces. Start reading the labels. You'll be unpleasantly surprised how much sugar you find where you least expect it. When you then consider the sugar-loaded foods most of us consume daily—soft drinks (the number-one source of sugar) and juice drinks, cakes, pies, cookies, frozen desserts, candy, and other snacks—it's easy to see how most of us eat about three to eight times the sugar we should. Fat-reduced prepared foods may even contain more sugar than their higher-fat counterparts.

How to Reduce Your Sugar Intake

Here's how to start cutting down today.

- **ELIMINATE THE "INVISIBLE" SUGARS FROM YOUR PANTRY AND REFRIGERATOR.** Read labels carefully and watch out for sugars you know (brown sugar, honey, molasses) and sugars by any other name: sucrose, glucose, maltose, fructose, corn syrup, corn sweetener, fruit juice concentrate, dextrose, invert sugar, and lactose.

- **EAT SMALL MEALS AND SNACKS THROUGHOUT THE DAY THAT INCLUDE SOME COMPLEX CARBOHYDRATES, SUCH AS WHOLE-GRAIN BREADS, STARCHY VEGETABLES, AND LEGUMES.** These nutrient-packed foods will promote a steady level of the brain chemical serotonin, which generally lifts your mood and reduces feelings of hunger.

- **NEVER SKIP BREAKFAST.** When you do, you're programming your body to crave sugar later in the morning.

- **PLAN YOUR SNACKS.** If you have a sweet tooth, don't defeat yourself by denying it. Instead, work into your daily diet a reasonable amount of sugar in foods that offer more, nutritionally speaking: flavored yogurt, fruit ices, and fig bars, for instance.

- **DON'T VILIFY THE SUGAR IN YOUR LIFE; JUST BE SURE YOU'RE EATING LESS OF IT.** One surefire way to spark a sugar binge is to outlaw it from your diet. Just be sensible instead. Cut back or eliminate sugar for a day or two and then enjoy that small slice of birthday cake at your daughter's party.

- **DRINK PLENTY OF WATER.** A desire for sugar, especially in the evening, can be a sign of thirst. Have a tall, cool glass of water—or two—and see how you feel before you grab that Oreo.

- **EXERCISE.** Even walking a few blocks or taking the stairs can boost your energy and short-circuit the sugar drive.

- **RELAX.** Stress and the hormones it produces often fuel sugar cravings. Be aware of what's really causing the craving, and try a few breathing exercises or other stress relievers before giving in.

- **DO IT GRADUALLY.** Begin by identifying and eliminating the sugar sources you can easily live without: "hidden sugars" in prepared foods, for instance, the candy dish on the coffee table, those cookies you keep around just in case you have guests. Every week, bring home one less sugar food from the store.

- **IDENTIFY THE SWEETS AND THE CIRCUMSTANCES THAT CAN TRIGGER A BINGE.** Don't bring home that apple pie or frozen German chocolate cake the week you know you'll be preparing the annual department review or inviting your seven-year-old's gymnastics class for a sleepover.

- **WATCH YOUR PORTIONS.** Experts point to ever-increasing serving sizes, such as the industrial-drum-size soft drinks sold at movie-theater concessions and fast-food restaurants. And warehouse and club shoppers, beware: Stocking the pantry with institutional quantities of anything makes them that much harder to resist. Of course, the lure is often getting more for your dollar, but ask yourself what you're really "saving"—maybe just those extra pounds. Instead of fretting about sweets going to waste, resolve that they're not going to your waist. If you're craving a special treat, buy just one.

100 CALORIES OF PLEASURE

1/4 cup premium ice cream
1 small candy bar
1/2 cup pudding
1/2 slice angel food cake with frosting
1/6 slice carrot cake with frosting
1/4 slice cheesecake
1/4 slice apple, blackberry, blueberry, cherry, or other fruit pie
1/4 slice lemon meringue pie
1/3 slice pumpkin pie
1/2 small package M&M's
4 large marshmallows
About 23 chocolate-covered raisins
1/3 cup sherbet

- **SAVE RICH DESSERTS FOR TRULY SPECIAL OCCASIONS.** And even then, get into the habit of sharing with your dinner partners. Remember, the fourth, eighth, and tenth bites really don't taste any better than the first.

- **INDULGE YOUR COMMON SENSE.** At about 50 calories a heaping tablespoon, whipped cream is just one of several dessert "accessories" that turn an exercise in moderation into something you really can feel guilty about. Forgo it, along with added syrups, nuts, and ice cream. Even with half the top layer of frosting set aside or half the pie crust left on the plate, most desserts lose none of their magic.

Take another look at high- and low-fat frozen yogurt and ice creams. Just remember: You may be better off with a serving of the real stuff that satisfies a craving than overdoing it on the low-fat versions.

ANOTHER LOOK AT LOW-FAT VERSUS LOW-CALORIE

the dessert, 1/2 cup	calories	protein gr.	fat gr.	calcium mg.
frozen vanilla yogurt, soft serve, sugar sweetened	114	2.8	4	102
vanilla ice cream, light, no sugar, sweetened with aspartame	98	2.9	4.2	127
vanilla ice cream, light, 50 percent fat of regular, sugar sweetened	91	2.5	2.8	91
vanilla ice cream, regular, sugar sweetened	132	2.3	7.2	84
vanilla ice cream, rich, sugar sweetened	178	2.6	12	86

IS YOUR DIET SODA UNDOING YOUR DIET?

Regular soft drinks are the epitome of empty calories, and switching to their artificially sweetened diet versions does eliminate those particular calories from your diet. But diet sodas have their downside too. Regular consumption of these fizzy, nutrition-free chemical brews can undermine your efforts to eat better, lose weight, and maintain your energy level. How? They make you feel hungrier and thirstier, and there is evidence that they whet your appetite for sweets but don't satisfy it, which makes that cookie look even better than it did before.

Here's a look at some of the villains found in diet sodas.

Aspartame (NutraSweet). The artificial sweetener that makes no-cal soda possible is a combination of two amino acids that can actually increase your craving for sugar and carbohydrates and your body's need for water. Also, a note to parents who believe NutraSweet is better for kids than sugar: It's not. In fact, aspartame is not recommended for children, especially young ones. One reason is a congenital condition called phenylketonuria (PKU), the inability to metabolize one of aspartame's amino acids, phenylalanine. In people with PKU (which affects about 1 in 20,000 babies), the unmetabolized phenylalanine builds up and causes mental retardation. Beyond that, a small percentage of people experience headache, dizziness, and epileptic-type seizures after ingesting aspartame. There's no question that aspartame can affect the brain; one study published in the esteemed British medical journal *Lancet* found that people with tinnitus found their symptoms were exacerbated by aspartame.

Phosphoric Acid. Phosphoric acid can deplete your body's levels of calcium and magnesium, reducing the amount of these minerals that stay in your blood and make it to your bones.

Sodium. This substance makes your body retain water.

Caffeine. Found in many diet and regular sodas, caffeine is a stimulant, which you may wish to avoid, and it also acts as a diuretic. We know that a body "starved" of water cannot function at top form, and one process that suffers is the ability to metabolize fat. Even worse, though, is the fact that increased urination takes with it B vitamins, calcium, and magnesium. Caffeine also prompts the pancreas to release insulin, which causes a blood-sugar surge followed by a drop that sets off hunger.

If you really can't give up soda, consider promoting it from a daily, habitual beverage to an occasional treat, and then really make it the real thing—with sugar, not aspartame. Juice-based carbonated drinks and carbonated, flavored bottled water or seltzer are good alternatives if you crave that fizz. "Juice drinks"—including Snapple, Fruitopia, and the like—are often high in sugar calories.

THIRTEEN "HEALTH" FOODS THAT AREN'T

Over the years, most of us have come to take on faith that certain health foods are either inherently very good for us or at least better than their unhealthy counterparts. Surprise! Here are thirteen foods that sound a lot healthier than they are.

1. **HONEY.** We're not so sweet on honey anymore. Offering hardly any nutrients and nearly a third more calories than sugar (63 per tablespoon to sugar's 46), honey's the better choice only if you prefer the taste. Think hard before adding it to your children's diet, since honey sticks tenaciously to teeth, which promotes cavities. And because honey may contain traces of botulism that could prove harmful, even fatal, to very young children, children under two should not have it.

2. **BEAN SPROUTS.** Low in fat, low in calories—and low in protein, vitamins, and minerals—bean sprouts have almost no nutritional value.

3. **EGGPLANT.** This vegetable got its place in the health food pantheon for its starring role in the classic vegetarian entrée eggplant Parmesan. Eggplant is low in nutrients, and when prepared with oil, it acts like a sponge. Ounce for ounce, fried eggplant is more fattening and less nutritious than french fries.

4. **VEGETABLE CHIPS.** In a rainbow of dusty oranges, pinks, and greens, veggie chips look so nutritious. After all, you reason, as you grab another handful, they *are* made from vegetables. But remember, so are their more honest cousins, good ol' potato chips. In fact, if you read most veggie-chip labels carefully, you'll find a smattering of carrot, beet, sweet potato (except for sweet potato chips), bell pepper, and other vegetable powders added to potato or corn. Processing kills most of the nutrients, and in the end, veggie chips are as high in fat and calories as regular potato or corn chips.

5. **GRANOLA.** Oats, nuts, fruit, honey—even the name sounds crunchy, sweet, and wholesome. So what's not to like about granola? Ounce for ounce, most regular granola contains as much sugar and fat as any high-sugar breakfast cereal and probably even more calories.

6. **"POWER" BARS.** True, most power bars pack a wallop in vitamins and minerals (which is one reason you should read the label before giving them to children; some bars contain levels of fat-soluble vitamins many times a child's RDA). But they also pack a lot of calories too. As for their protein content, you probably eat more than enough protein already. (See "Protein: Pro and Con," page 131.)

7. **"WHOLE-GRAIN," "ORGANIC" BAKED GOODS AND DESSERTS.** A calorie is a calorie, no matter what it comes in. There's nothing wrong with the occasional

dessert, but don't add, "And it's good for me," to your list of reasons for going for seconds.

8. **NONDAIRY DESSERT AND PUDDING SUBSTITUTES (TOFUTTI, RICE DREAM, ET AL.).** These products are godsends for people who choose not to eat dairy products. However, you have to read the labels. Tofutti, for example, contains a high percentage of fat, and there's no savings in calories if you compare a cup of Rice Dream pudding to the regular stuff.

9. **WRAP SANDWICHES.** If the tortilla is more than 6 inches wide, the wrap probably has more calories than it should. Go for low-fat cheese and lean-meat fillings. Veggies are great too, but avoid roasted vegetables, which may be swimming in oil. Ask for your wrap prepared with a low-fat or fat-free spread, rather than oil, mayonnaise, butter, or guacamole.

10. **BOTTLED HEALTH JUICES.** The exotic names, such as Passion Fruit Energizer, are attractive, and with a smattering of vitamins and minerals thrown in, they are slightly superior to other bottled juices. But not by much. Most health juices contain only about 5 to 25 percent fruit juice (for comparison's sake, Hi-C contains 5 percent fruit juice); the rest is water and some form of sugar. With calorie content ranging as high as 400 for 20 ounces, you might consider getting your vitamins from your food and supplements and drinking whole juice or water instead.

11. **FRUIT AND FROZEN SHAKES, SMOOTHIES.** They're made from fresh fruit, low-fat frozen yogurt, and usually additional sweetener, and they look, smell, and taste delicious. But they are not the troves of nutrients you might think, and if your fruits are juiced, they lose the fiber that would make you feel full.

12. **TRAIL MIX AND DRIED-FRUIT/NUT SNACKS.** Yes, they're "natural," but they're also chock-full of calories and, with nuts, fat. Nuts average 150 to 200 calories per ounce, raisins about 50, and dried coconut over 100. And when it comes to promoting cavities, dried fruits are worse than candy because they cling to the teeth.

13. **PREPARED "ORGANIC" OR "NATURAL" FOODS.** Once inside the health food store, many of us stop reading labels, which is a big mistake. You may be surprised to discover that soy macaroni and cheese contains just as much fat and

as many calories as regular macaroni and cheese, for example, or that many frozen entrées contain high levels of fat, not to mention many calories.

EAT SOMETHING: YOU'LL FEEL BETTER

By now we all know the basics of eating for optimal mood and performance:

- a good breakfast that combines carbohydrates and protein;

- complex-carbohydrate, low-fat, no-junk snacking;

- some protein at lunch;

- a moderate, healthy dinner;

- healthy snacking as needed to even out energy dips.

And, of course, we all need exercise.

In addition, there are foods, beverages, spices, vitamins, and minerals with proven powers to soothe, comfort, or even cure a range of problems.

If you experience . . .	try . . .	because . . .
mild depression and PMS	banana	B_6 helps regulate blood glucose levels, which can affect mood.
insomnia	banana	the high carbohydrate content will boost the effectiveness of tryptophan in our bodies, which helps us sleep.
mild depression and irritability	spinach	B_9 (folic acid) has been shown to help improve these symptoms.
insomnia and mild anxiety	milk and other dairy products	calcium may alleviate these symptoms.

If you experience . . .	try . . .	because . . .
generally down moods	hot peppers	capsaicin, the chemical that puts the "hot" in hot peppers, stimulates the brain to produce the "feel good" neurochemicals known as endorphins.
mild depression, irritability, anxiety, and insomnia	almonds	calcium and magnesium found in almonds enable our bodies to better deal with stress.
stress	red bell peppers	stress depletes vitamin C, which 1/2 cup red bell peppers can more than restore—158 percent of your RDA.
headache	caffeinated coffee, tea, soft drinks	caffeine, long a staple in many over-the-counter headache remedies, constricts overly widened blood vessels in the head, which may cause headaches. There is a lot of bad press about caffeine, and it should be ingested in moderation, like everything else. But it can be a more effective headache remedy than aspirin, Tylenol, or Aleve, and it's perfectly safe unless you're especially sensitive to it.
gout	cherries, cherry juice	cherries contain several minerals—including potassium, calcium, phosphorus, magnesium, manganese, copper, and iron—that have a positive effect on collagen metabolism and the body's ability to reduce inflammation.

If you experience . . .	try . . .	because . . .
nasal congestion	hot mustards or Japanese-type horseradish	mustard and horseradish, added to food, are natural decongestants.
toothache	cloves	2 whole cloves held in the mouth whole or chewed can temporarily numb toothache pain.
tension	chew gum or a crunchy food such as carrots; or snack on high-carb foods such as rice cakes and crunchy fruit	chewing increases blood flow and releases muscular tension; eating carbohydrates boosts serotonin, which improves mood and may make it easier for some people to eat in moderation.
migraine headache	ginger	ginger has anti-inflammatory qualities; a "tea" made of 1/3 teaspoon ground ginger in water, taken three to four times a day, can circumvent a migraine headache if taken when the first symptoms occur. Do not use ginger if you are or may be pregnant or have had or plan to have surgery within a few days.

ARE YOU EATING ENOUGH TO LOSE WEIGHT?

If that strikes you as an odd question, it's because we've all been brainwashed into believing we can't shed pounds without starving on 1,200 or fewer calories a day. True, there are some people who can function well in their daily lives (by which I mean they are not exhausted, irritable, and confused) and lose weight on 1,200 calories. But if you currently weigh over 100 pounds and are moderately active, you probably are not one of them.

As anyone who's endured a low-calorie, quick (as in more than 2 pounds per week) weight-loss diet can attest, once the diet's "over," the quick weight-regain-phase kicks in with a vengeance. That's because your body is too smart to let you lose too much weight too quickly. Through slowing your metabolism and making you feel ravenously hungry, your body will fight to restore the equilibrium. Anyone who's losing more than 2 pounds a week is probably losing more water than fat. The fat we do break down is flooding our systems with its long-stored cache of toxins, which can leave you with headaches and an overall miserable feeling. Between carrying us through our daily lives on fewer calories than we need and coping with toxin overload, our bodies can't help but respond with fatigue, depression, and cravings.

You may be amazed to learn that a 140-pound moderately active person can lose a pound a week on 1,500 calories a day. For a 180-pound person, make that 2,000. With the right food choices and exercise, you can both feed your body and starve your fat cells (which beats starving your body and killing your diet any day).

TRY EASING INTO A NEW WAY OF EATING

If you've had trouble sticking to a reduced-calorie eating plan before, try easing your way into it. Instead of starting off cutting 500 calories a day, cut 100 a day the first week, 200 a day the second week, and so on. While you probably won't lose much weight during those first weeks, you may do better in the long run.

Getting to Work (Out)

3.

. . . .

Helene began working out with me about a year ago. When I met her, she was in her mid-thirties, about 30 pounds overweight, and had not really paid much attention to her health over the past five years. She was intelligent and concerned about her health and her appearance, but something always seemed to stand between her and her goals. That first day, she sat across from me, shoulders stooped, head down, and said quietly, "I'm just fat and self-conscious about it. I know I have to do something, but I can't bear the thought of working out around other people. I can't stand the way I look." Helene and I agreed that she would start training with me, in private sessions, three times a week.

Over the next few months, I saw a remarkable change in Helene.

Not only did she lose 25 pounds and essentially reshape and tone her body—which was amazing enough—but she became a new woman. It was as if with every pound she dropped, every new routine she mastered, something inside of her came forward. She walked with confidence now; when she spoke, she looked you in the eye. She told me she felt calmer, more energetic, and happier. In terms of her progress at the gym, it looked as if there was nothing she couldn't do.

HOW MUCH EXERCISE IS ENOUGH?

Too many people approach an "exercise program" as an all-or-nothing proposition. They fall victim to a pervasive, self-defeating, and medically inaccurate belief that they aren't "really" working out unless they devote at least an hour every day to a draining session in a high-tech gym, climbing a fake cliff or pressing twice their body weight. Since most of us can't, won't, or don't want to do this, we may just give up on exercise altogether. Don't. And don't rationalize your sedentary lifestyle with the belief that eating well, avoiding stress, and staying trim are enough to keep you fit. Here's the shocking truth: Failure to exercise regularly is as debilitating to your health as smoking.

The good news is that you needn't be perfectly sculpted, buffed, and cut to be physically fit. The key is a program of moderate exercise that meets the surgeon general's recommendation: Thirty minutes or more of physical activity on most or all days. It sounds like a modest goal, but the positive results are impressive. You can:

- reduce your risk of osteoporosis, heart disease, some forms of cancer (namely, breast, uterine, ovarian, and colorectal), and non-insulin-dependent diabetes;

- reduce your blood cholesterol;

- control your blood pressure;

- improve your mood and ability to cope with everyday stress;

- safely lose weight;

- increase your energy and improve your emotional health;

- improve your resistance to disease;

- get a better night's sleep.

The fact that moderate exercise usually carries little risk of exercise-related injury is another plus. If you have or are at risk for any chronic health problem (for example, heart disease, diabetes, obesity, or high blood pressure), consult with your physician before you begin.

Not surprisingly, the most popular form of moderate exercise is brisk walking. It can be easily incorporated into even the busiest schedule, has low injury rates, does not require any special skill or equipment, and can be done by anyone at any age. But walking isn't the only beneficial activity, and you might be surprised to realize how many other "exercise opportunities" daily living affords. Gardening, waxing the car, and running the vacuum all help improve muscle strength. Obviously, you need to spend less time at more intense activity levels, more time at less intense ones.

So, if you can't make that thirty-minute walk today, here are some other ways that may contribute to meeting your daily exercise quotient.

WALKING OR RUNNING WITH WEIGHTS?

Don't. True, you do have to exert more effort to walk or run holding light free weights or wearing weight bands. So it seems logical that the extra effort would burn more calories and tone arms and upper body. Surprisingly, however, walking with weights has exactly the opposite effect. Swinging your arms in a vigorous, controlled manner burns 10 percent to 15 percent of the total calories expended by walking, jogging, or running. People who add weights generally don't move their arms and upper body as much, and the small amount of toning they may derive from carrying the weights isn't enough to offset what they've lost in terms of calories burned and upper-body movement.

WHAT CONSTITUTES "MODERATE EXERCISE"?

ACTIVITY	DURATION/ MINUTES	
Washing and waxing a car	45 to 60	
Washing windows or floors	45 to 60	
Playing volleyball	45	
Playing touch football	30 to 45	
Gardening	30 to 45	
Wheeling yourself in a manual wheelchair	30 to 40	
Walking	35	1¼ miles, 20 minutes/mile
Basketball, shooting baskets	30	
Bicycling, brisk	30	5 miles, 6 minutes/mile
Dancing fast, social	30	
Pushing a stroller	30	1½ miles, 20 minutes/mile
Raking leaves	30	
Water aerobics	30	
Swimming laps	20	
Playing wheelchair basketball	20	

WHAT CONSTITUTES "MODERATE EXERCISE"? *(continued)*

ACTIVITY	DURATION/ MINUTES	
Playing a game of basketball	*15 to 20*	
Bicycling, leisurely	*30*	*4 miles, 7½ minutes/mile*
Jumping rope	*15*	
Running	*15*	*1½ miles, 10 minutes/mile*
Shoveling snow	*15*	
Stair walking	*15*	

Exercise Reminders

Yes, we exercise to get in shape, but there are forms of exercise you need to be in shape for. Nothing short-circuits our resolve to exercise faster than an injury or coming home sore. No matter what physical activity you engage in—whether it's moving furniture or running a marathon—always:

- warm up first and cool down afterward, even if you're just tossing a Frisbee;

- drink enough water before, during, and after;

- stop at the first sign of pain or injury;

- perform aerobic workouts with a certified (ACE or ACSM) instructor;

- stick to activities you have the strength and endurance to perform;

- wear the right clothing and shoes, use the best form, and observe basic safety precautions at all times.

A STITCH IN TIME

Sooner or later, nearly everyone who exercises gets that gnawingly sharp, seemingly endless pain in the side commonly known as a stitch. Few of us mind being in stitches when something strikes us as funny, but when stitches hit during a workout or even yard work, it's no laughing matter. Most of us slow down or stop, try to breathe (which isn't always easy), and just get the darn thing to go away.

Stitches can be very painful, because they are cramps that occur when the large muscles between the ribs and the diaphragm go into spasm. Muscles go into spasm when the body fails to meet their demand for oxygen. The harder your muscles are working, the more oxygen they need. The secret to preventing stitches is to gradually raise your body's core temperature and increase blood flow to your muscles before your workout begins.

To Avoid Getting a Stitch

- Make sure you warm up thoroughly before you begin exercising. You can warm up effectively by doing your regular workout but at a slower, less strenuous pace. If you'll be doing aerobics, run through them at a more leisurely pace. Runners might jog first; cyclists might pedal but at a slower pace, perhaps in a lower gear. Follow the aerobic portion of your warmup with deliberate, controlled stretching of the muscles you'll be using. Doing your stretches after you've warmed up aerobically protects against injury by making the muscles warmer and more flexible.

- Work out at lower intensity for a longer period of time.

- If you are increasing the intensity of your workout, do it gradually. And if during your workout you "shift gears" from a low-level activity to a higher one, take a few moments to warm up to the next phase.

- If you're prone to getting stitches after meals, wait thirty to ninety minutes after you eat to exercise.

An exercise program that burns the optimum number of calories will include five thirty- to forty-five-minute sessions per week working within your target heart rate (THR) zone. If you can't fit in five sessions a week, don't worry. Obviously, the more you can do, the greater your benefit. When it comes to cardiovascular workouts, however, even once a week is better than nothing.

Measuring your heart rate—the number of times your heart beats per minute—is one way to be sure that you're exercising at the right pace. At the low end of the THR zone, you're barely sweating; at the high end, you're really working. If you're a beginner, stick to the lower end so that you can exercise for longer periods of time each session. As you become more fit, you can train in the middle and upper end of your THR zone. If you find that you're doing the same workout but not achieving as high a target heart rate as you did before, it may mean that your cardiovascular fitness has improved. Your heart is stronger, so it doesn't need to beat as many times per minute as it did before. You should continue your workout, but increase the intensity to keep your heart rate in the high end of your target heart rate zone. However, never exceed 90 percent of your maximum heart rate.

Determine Your THR Zone

Here's how to determine your target heart rate zone. Keep in mind that this formula can give you only an estimate, a basic range.

1. Find your estimated maximum heart rate (MHR) by subtracting your age from 220.

2. Multiply the MHR number from step 1 by 50%, or 0.50. This will give you the lower end of your THR zone.

3. Multiply your MHR number again (from step 1), this time by 85%, or 0.85. This will give you the higher end of your THR zone.

For example, if you are forty-two years old, your math would look like this:

1. $220 - 42 = 178$ (the estimated maximum heart rate)

2. $178 \times 0.50 = 89$ (the lower end of your THR zone)

3. $178 \times 0.85 = 151$ (the higher end of your THR zone)

If you're forty-two, then, your target heart rate zone is 89 (lower end) to 151 (higher end). If your heart beats fewer than 89 times per minute, you're not pushing hard enough. If it beats more than 151 times per minute, slow down.

TARGET HEART RATE ZONES, BY AGE	
Age	*Beats per Minute*
25	98–146
30	95–142
40	90–135
45	88–131

How to Check Your Heart Rate While Working Out

During your workout, you can take your heart rate at fifteen-minute intervals. Place your index finger and your middle finger on the side of your neck between your ear and your shoulder. When you feel a beat, you've found your carotid artery. While looking at the second hand of a clock or watch, count the beats for ten seconds. Multiply the number of beats by 6. This tells you how many times your heart beats per minute and where it is in relation to your THR zone. The specificity of the THR gives you an objective measure of your workout. If you keep a record of your workouts to chart your progress, the THR comes in very handy.

PERCEIVED EXERTION

Another easy way to determine the intensity of your workout is perceived exertion. This method uses a numerical scale from 1 to 10 that corresponds to how hard you perceive you're working. Perceived exertion and your THR are both valid ways to make sure you're exercising at the right pace.

PERCEIVED EXERTION SCALE

number	rating	sample activities
0	zero	sitting, watching television
I	very light	sitting, reading a magazine
2	light	standing in grocery-store line
3	light	grocery shopping
4	light/moderate	gardening
5	moderate	walking at a leisurely pace
6	moderate/hard	jogging briskly
7	hard	hiking
8	very hard	running
9	harder	running uphill
10	extremely hard	chopping wood

SUBMAXIMAL TEST

Finally, if you have been exercising at the high end of your THR zone and feel that your workout is no longer challenging, ask your doctor to perform a submaximal test. This test evaluates your heart rate while you're working to about 75 percent to 85 percent of your maximum, on a treadmill. The test usually takes fifteen minutes or more. During this time, the intensity is increased every three or four minutes while the doctor monitors your heart rate and blood pressure. This is the most accurate measure of your aerobic capacity. After you have your test results, talk to your doctor about your exercise program.

WHY BODY TYPE MATTERS

You may not know which type of exercise is best for you, but your body does. When it comes to exercise, one size most definitely does not fit all. That's because body types are born, not made. And while the right exercise program can bring out the best in any body type, no amount of exercise can change your basic shape. The goal of following the right exercise program for your body type is summed up in the old song: "Accentuate the Positive."

The first step is to determine your body type. Look at the four basic types listed below and see which description best fits your body. When you think of how your body weight is distributed, consider both muscle and fat. If, following a period of exercising for one body type, a new body type "emerges"—for example, if sensible eating and exercise bring out the hourglass that used to look like a pear—modify your workout to fit. But don't embark on a fitness program with a specific body type as your goal. I've seen too many people give up on exercise when, after doing the wrong exercises for their body type, they are disappointed that they haven't morphed into a totally new shape. They may inadvertently end up with a bigger rear end or a disproportionately large upper body. Remember: You can improve on your body type, but it's impossible to change it.

THE BASIC FOUR BODY TYPES

1. **HOURGLASS.** Even if you're not the classic—and for most women, physiologically impossible—36–24–36, you can make the most of having been born with relatively equal upper- and lower-body proportions. Your goal should be to maintain your proportions.
   RECOMMENDED PROGRAM: Invest equal strength-training time in working the upper and lower body, using light (3 to 5 pounds) to moderate (8 to 12 pounds) weights and doing more repetitions (20 to 50). Avoid working out with heavy weights.

2. **LEAN.** With a fat-distribution pattern that spreads itself equally instead of concentrated in one area, women with a lean body type often appear not to have "problem areas," but they may lack muscle strength.

RECOMMENDED PROGRAM: High- and low-intensity aerobics and strength training, three times a week, with extra attention to abdominals if they're weak.

3. **PEAR.** If you're among the 75 percent of American women whose fat deposits on the bottom and thighs, your objective will be to reduce lower-body mass while building the upper body to create more balanced proportions.

RECOMMENDED PROGRAM: High-intensity, low-resistance aerobics of long duration four times a week, such as running. Strength training twice a week will tone muscles. High-impact aerobics, such as incline walking, jogging, running, and step classes, will increase muscle mass exactly where you're trying to reduce—so avoid them. For strength training, go for light (3 to 5 pounds) weights with more repetitions (20 to 50) to strengthen the lower body without adding unwanted mass. To build the upper body, go for moderate to heavy (10 to 15 pounds) weights.

4. **APPLE.** This body type is marked by a tendency to store fat in the abdomen, tops of hips, and waist, so that arms and legs appear disproportionately thin compared to the torso.

RECOMMENDED PROGRAM: Try to work out four or five times a week, alternating a longer medium-intensity session (45 minutes to an hour) with a briefer high-intensity session (30 minutes). Your goal is to burn fat while building your upper and lower body with light (3 to 5 pounds) to moderate (8 to 12 pounds) weights, performing strength work. The "Superman Lift" (see page 235) is great for toning the midsection.

FOUR ESSENTIAL EXERCISES FOR GREAT LEGS

No matter what your body type, firm, shapely legs not only look great, they feel great too. Whether you want to have the legs miniskirts were made for or relieve tired, achy legs and possibly ward off varicose and spider veins, here are four effective, universal moves anyone can benefit from. (Note: Do not do these if you have knee or back problems.)

The Lunge

1. Stand with your feet pointing forward, shoulder width apart, your back straight. Look straight ahead.

2. While bending at the knee, step forward with your right foot, all the while keeping your knee aligned over your big toe. Do not bend so deeply that your knee extends beyond your toe. Your left leg should be straight and you should be standing on the ball of your left foot.

3. Using the muscles in your front, lunging leg (the right), return to the starting position. Remember not to use your left leg to "help" with this move. All the work should be done by the lunging leg.

4. Alternate legs, lunging with your left leg forward, your right leg behind.

5. Repeat for eight lunges on each side.

Thigh Toner

1. Lie flat on the floor. Tilt your pelvis up so that your lower back touches the floor.

2. Slowly lift both of your legs so that they form a 90-degree angle with the floor. Place your hands under your lower back for support.

3. Slowly open and close your legs in a controlled scissoring motion.

4. Do three sets of eight "scissors."

Hip and Hamstring Firmer

1. Stand behind the back of a chair, with your feet shoulder width apart. Place your hands on the chair for balance. Don't lock your knees.

2. Without arching your back, extend your right leg behind you. Be careful not to lock your knee or kick your leg out behind you. This should be a very slow, controlled lifting motion.

3. Do eight extensions with your right leg; alternate for eight with the left. Continue alternating until you've done three sets of eight reps with each leg.

Calf Firmer

1. Stand with your feet flat on the floor, shoulder width apart, and your toes pointing slightly outward.

2. Holding the top of a chair for balance, rise up as high as you can on your toes. Be sure your torso remains straight up and down. Hold for a count of five and slowly return to the starting position. Do not bounce or move quickly.

3. Do three sets of eight reps. *Advanced move:* Do one leg at a time.

WHAT CAN I DO ABOUT WATER RETENTION IN MY LEGS?

Massage it away in about three minutes! Massage not only stimulates circulation and improves muscle tone, it also prevents fluid accumulation in your legs. Another plus: Your legs are one of the few areas of your body you can self-massage effectively. Also remember to sit or lie with your legs elevated to at least hip level for ten minutes or more a day.

1. Stand or sit with your legs extended. Apply a warmed body oil.
2. Using a long kneading stroke, and starting from the ankles and working up, lift your muscles and work them back and forth. Push in opposite directions with both hands.
3. Once you've massaged your whole leg, apply several slow, firm, deep strokes from the ankle up.

RECLAIM YOUR RIGHT TO BARE ARMS

Jiggly arms, batwings—call them what you will. Those droopy upper-arm muscles—biceps at the front, triceps at the back—are enough to keep most of us in long sleeves all summer long. And that's a shame, because just three half-hour strength-training sessions a week can make a big difference in the shape, tone, and strength of the muscles, and can also help your body burn calories more efficiently. In as little as three to four weeks, you will see the positive results of weight training, particularly in the upper body, because you are working a number of small-muscle groups. Not only will your arms be firmer and stronger, your toned-up shoulders will actually make your hips appear smaller! What other incentive do you need? And these exercises are great for all body types.

- If you're a beginner, start with 3-pound hand-held free weights, or dumbbells. At these weights, you should feel challenged but not strained. When you can complete your routine with little effort, it's time to bump up the weight in 1- to 2-pound increments. Note, however, that beyond 10 pounds you should be working with a spotter. Frankly, there's no reason to move up to a higher weight unless you're seriously into weight training.

- Do each exercise through the entire "range of motion"—that is, to the fullest extent the joint allows without pain or discomfort.

- If the exercise calls for you to stand, be sure to always: (1) keep your feet hip width apart, toes pointing forward, with your knees slightly bent (do not lock your knees!); and (2) tighten your abdominal muscles and tuck your pelvis under to stabilize your back.

- Be sure every movement is slow and controlled. Don't let your arms "fly" out from your sides. Lift the weights, don't "swing" them.

- Work conscientiously, making sure that you really concentrate on the muscles you're working.

- Before you start, always warm up at least five minutes. This raises your body's core temperature and stimulates circulation. You don't need a special "routine."

Anything that gets your blood flowing is great: walking, stair climbing, or using an exercise bike or treadmill.

- After you finish your routine, spend five minutes stretching.

Lying One-Arm Extension (Triceps)

1. Lie on your back with your legs bent, feet pressed firmly onto the floor. Hold a dumbbell in your right hand beside you, with your palm facing toward your body.

2. Extend the arm facing you straight up toward the ceiling. Support with your free hand through the following steps.

3. Bend your arm at the elbow, and lower the dumbbell back toward the side of your head.

4. Slowly straighten your arm. Repeat up to eight times total, then switch to the left arm. Start with one set of eight, and then work up to three sets of eight reps on each side.

Hammer Curl (Biceps)

1. Sit in a chair with a dumbbell in each hand, palm facing toward the side of your body. (Hold it the same way you would hold a suitcase.)

2. Bending your arm at the elbow, lift the dumbbell toward your shoulder, keeping your upper arm and elbow close to your body. Do not let your elbows "fly." Hold for five seconds.

3. Slowly lower the dumbbell back to the starting position, then repeat exercise with your left arm. Alternate sides for eight reps. Gradually work up to three sets of eight reps.

Biceps Curl (Biceps)

1. Sit in a chair with a dumbbell in each hand, palm facing toward you.

2. With your right arm, lift the dumbbell toward your right shoulder, keeping your elbow close to your body. Hold five seconds.

3. Slowly lower the dumbbell back to starting position, then repeat exercise with your left arm. Alternate sides for eight reps. Gradually work up to three sets of eight reps.

FOUR MINUTES TO TIGHT ABS

Your abdominal muscles—or abs—occupy the front of your torso, from the thorax to the pelvis. Good, solid abs are the foundation of a healthy body. If you think of your abdominal area as the center of your body, the juncture where your upper body and arms and lower body and legs meet, it's easy to understand the abs' importance. Toned abdominals not only give you better posture and better balance, they also provide a strong "base" that supports your body through the countless motions of daily living, not to mention exercise and sports activities.

Weak abdominals produce more than tight-fitting waistbands. Abdominals that can't carry their weight in front wreak havoc on the back too. Every year, Americans spend over $50 billion on medical care for problems related to lower back pain. For most of them, back problems are chronic, lifelong, and debilitating. In most cases, medical intervention is temporary and unsatisfactory, so it makes sense to prevent back problems before they start. And if a future trip to the chiropractor or orthopedist isn't incentive enough, remember: Beach season comes every year.

Where, Exactly, Are the Abs?

It's easy to identify the group of four muscles known collectively as the abs when you know what they do.

1. **TRANSVERSUS ABDOMINIS.** When you suck in your stomach, this is the deep muscle you tighten.

2. **RECTUS ABDOMINIS.** This sheath of muscles that stretches between your sternum and your pubic bone helps you bend forward.

3. **EXTERNAL OBLIQUES.** Each set runs at an angle from the lower ribs to the front of the hip bone, forming an incomplete V that fans downward. These are the muscles you use whenever you twist your body, flex your spine, or bend to the side.

4. **INTERNAL OBLIQUES.** These criss-cross and work in conjunction with the external obliques to make the above motions possible.

Of course, there's much more to know about all of these amazing muscles, but this is all you need to know to get to work.

For every exercise, remember:

- to inhale while resting and exhale during the crunch;

- to be sure you're isolating and working only your abdominal muscles;

- to not "pull yourself up" by your head, neck, or arms. If you feel your neck or upper back begin to tighten, lie back, breathe deeply, and relax;

- to always move in a smooth, controlled motion. With abs it's the quality of the movement, not its size or speed, that determines its effectiveness. Forget the jerky, full sit-ups you learned in gym class;

- to not relax your abs upon returning to the start position, unless otherwise instructed.

Abdominal Crunch

1. Lie on your back with your calves resting on a bench, chair, or couch so that your legs are bent at a 90-degree angle. Your knees should be directly over your hips.

2. Relax your hips and let your knees and feet open naturally and comfortably. This "deactivates" other muscles (the hip flexors) and helps you isolate your abdominals.

3. Tighten your abdominals so that your lower spine straightens enough to make contact with the floor.

4. Cross your arms over your chest with your fingertips touching the opposite shoulder. In the correct position, you'll be able to rest your chin on your wrists for support. Lift your elbows slightly so they point at your knees.

5. Now the crunch: In one controlled motion, simultaneously lift your upper torso, shoulders, head, and neck. (As you rise, think of rising from the lowest body part through the highest. This will help you avoid "leading" or "pulling" with your neck.) Go up and forward in two counts until your shoulder blades clear the floor; exhale through the second count. While it may seem you haven't lifted yourself very high, this is as far as you can go and still be working the abdominals. If you go any further, your hip flexors will be assuming the bulk of the work.

6. Slowly lower your back to the starting position without relaxing your abdominals, then repeat for a total of four sets of eight reps.

The Twist

1. Lie down, with calves elevated, in the position described in steps 1 through 3 of the previous exercise. Place your left hand on the outside of your left thigh for support, but be sure you're not using it to pull yourself up. Place your right hand behind your head so that your thumb is resting behind your right ear and your fingers are spread for support. Again, make sure you are not pulling your head and neck up with your hand.

2. Lift your head and torso up and forward as you did in the crunch. After your shoulders have cleared the floor, twist your right shoulder toward your left knee. Try to imagine a straight line running from your left knee to your right shoulder pulling them together. Be careful not to use your hips to twist. Do one set of eight reps.

3. Return to the starting position without relaxing your abdominals. Change the position of your hands (so your right hand is on your right thigh, your left hand behind your head), and repeat on the other side. Do one set of eight reps. Work up to four sets of eight reps per side.

Reverse Curl

1. Begin from the start position described in "The Twist" above. But this time, place your hands flat on the floor at your sides, near your hips, so that your arms can provide balance.

2. On the count of one, in a slow, controlled movement, bring your knees into your chest while keeping your knees together.

3. Visualize your abdominals pulling toward your spine as you contract them while slightly lifting your hips off the floor until your buttocks and tailbone are clear.

4. Over two counts, return to the starting position, and without relaxing your abdominals, repeat for four sets of eight reps.

NEW WAYS TO EXERCISE

When asked why they quit or never committed themselves to exercise, many people say, "I got bored." Integrating exercise into your life is not easy, and excuses can be tempting. Before boredom with your current routine creeps in and undoes all your good work, consider trying something new, different, and exciting. Don't wait until you're ready to quit to spice up your fitness repertoire with one—or maybe even all—of these.

Are You Ready to Sweat?

• If you're already in good shape with a high level of cardiovascular fitness and aerobic capacity, you might try increasing the intensity and duration of your workout.

- For all the cardio-intensive punch with a lot less impact, go for spinning—an intensive stationary-cycling class borrowed from pro-cycling training. Here an instructor puts you through your paces.

- Kickboxing—includes jumping rope, punching bags, weight training, and shadow boxing—all of which will improve your endurance, sharpen your reflexes, get your heart going, and strengthen your muscles.

- You don't need a beach or the summer sun to get all the cardiovascular and muscle-toning benefits of volleyball. Indoor sandpits make it a year-round activity.

Give Your Mind a Little Workout Too

- Rock climbing on man-made climbing walls presents both mental and physical challenges. You can build strong, well-sculpted muscles (especially in your arms) while scaling the course and finding your next hand- and toeholds.

- Though martial art forms differ in philosophy and the type of physical activity involved, all regard the student's mental powers as being as important as her physical prowess in executing its *katas,* or movements. Tae kwon do and karate involve punches, kicks, and other defensive techniques. Judo and kung fu involve more hand-to-hand combat. All require intensive mental discipline, which some people find they carry into other aspects of their lives.

Deceptively Subtle, Yet Effective

- Hatha yoga is an ancient Indian technique that uses posture, movement, and breathing to increase overall health, relaxation, flexibility, and strength. Yoga is recommended for people who cannot participate in high-impact activities or who want to learn to get more in touch with their bodies. Hatha is only one of many types of yoga. Others may place a greater emphasis on yoga's spiritual aspects or involve very intensive physical activity. Be sure to find out what your instructor has in mind before you begin.

- Pilates is an exercise program developed early in this century by Joseph Pilates. Because Pilates improves posture, flexibility, and coordination while at the same time building muscles that are stronger but not bulkier, it's been the favorite of dancers for decades. People who want a total-body workout without stressing their joints should try this. Pilates movements must be executed with precision; no zoning out here. Some exercises involve special machines, unique to the method, and the close supervision of a specially trained Pilates instructor is crucial to the program's success. Pilates instructors can be found in most major cities, and gyms are beginning to offer classes with trained instructors.

- Tai chi looks like a slow-motion version of another martial art, but in fact it's much more. Tai chi is actually a form of active meditation that's been practiced in China for centuries. It develops balance and flexibility. And while it is not considered aerobically intense, a recent pilot study by the American Heart Association found that older people who practiced tai chi showed a decrease in blood pressure nearly as great as that of a group enrolled in a moderately intense aerobics class.

Have Fun

- Dancing—whether it's jazz, tap, square, line, swing, ballet, hip-hop, done solo or with a partner or partners—is great exercise. In addition to offering a cardiovascular workout, dance develops coordination, timing, flexibility, and good posture.

- Hiking is a great reason to get outdoors. It helps develop cardiovascular endurance and tones the lower body.

WHEN TO EXERCISE

If exercise is so good for you, any time is the right time, right? Maybe not. People who have an established exercise routine usually discover, through trial and error, a time of day when their workout feels easier, more invigorating, and more fun. If you exercise at different times each day and/or your workout leaves you feeling more worked over than anything else, you might want to rethink your approach.

Like every other species on the planet, we all have internal biological "clocks" that determine the circadian rhythms of our body's many systems. We all know those times of day when we're most alert or most likely to nap, those periods when it's easiest to fall asleep, think creatively, or be patient with our kids or the boss. Body temperature, sleep cycle, metabolism, and blood pressure are just a few of the biological processes regulated and "scheduled" by the hypothalamus, a gland located in the brain.

Scientists have found that variations in body temperature can directly enhance or diminish exercise performance. Simply put, the higher your body temperature, the better your muscles perform, and the more productive and satisfying your workout. Warm, flexible muscles are stronger, quicker, and less likely to be injured. For most people, late afternoon is when body temperature peaks; one to three hours before you wake in the morning is when it dips the lowest (which is why warming up is especially crucial for morning exercising).

A late-afternoon workout isn't feasible for everyone, and some who try it find it makes no difference in how they feel. Even though, theoretically, the early-morning workout should be the most challenging, people who start their day with exercise may find it easier to stay committed to their program, perhaps because nothing else is competing for their attention. And they get the satisfaction of knowing they've done their exercise for the day.

A TIME TO TRAIN

No matter when you usually work out, if you're training for an upcoming event, such as a marathon, you will perform better if you train at the same time of day the event will be held.

DON'T LET YOUR AFTER-WORKOUT SHOWER DRY YOU OUT

A relaxing, hot shower after a good, hard workout. Ah . . . Try uh-oh. Your elevated body temperature combined with the heat of a hot shower may result in dehydration, dizziness, or weakness. Cool down from your cool down. Wait five to ten minutes before taking a refreshing shower in lukewarm water.

FUEL YOUR WORKOUT

When you engage in any physical activity, your muscles use glycogen, a form of sugar. The body can't make glycogen without glucose, can't make glucose without protein and carbohydrates, and can't get either of the latter if you don't eat. Working out depletes the glycogen stored in your muscles, and it takes about a day for it to be replaced. Here are the best ways to eat to maximize your morning, midday, or evening workout and ensure that your muscles will be fully "fueled" for tomorrow too.

- **MORNING.** To counteract a low-rising blood-sugar level, try to eat something light—fruit, yogurt, toast, cereal—about half an hour before your morning workout. The first two hours after your workout is peak time for your body to resynthesize glycogen, so be sure to eat within that time.

- **MIDDAY.** Depending on when you ate breakfast, you should snack an hour or so before your midday workout. If you don't, your blood sugar will be very low. Be sure to eat within two hours of your workout.

- **EVENING.** Some people find that working out at night makes it difficult for them to sleep. Working out in the early evening, though, has some great advantages: diminished appetite and faster metabolism. Ideally, you should have a light snack about two hours before you exercise, then a light dinner after.

And always make sure you drink plenty of water, before, during, and after any workout.

Foods That Can Slow You Down

- Rich, fatty foods, because they take longer to digest;

- Salty foods, because they cause your body to retain water;

- Carbonated beverages, because they give you a quick sugar surge and they can make you feel bloated;

- No-calorie snacks (such as raw vegetables), because they are hard to digest and they provide no energy;

- Candy (including high-calorie "sports" bars), because they cause a rapid rise in blood sugar followed by a sudden crash.

HOW CAN SPORTS DRINKS NOT BE GOOD FOR YOU?

First, sports drinks were originally formulated to meet the immediate calorie needs of athletes engaged in high-intensity activities. This is why they're high in sugar, calories, and sodium, none of which most of us really need, no matter how vigorously we work out. Some people find that the sudden sugar rush leaves them with a headache. And no sports drink is as thirst quenching as water. Before you grab a sports drink for yourself or a child, also consider this: Researchers at the University of Liverpool's School of Dentistry found that, like fruit juices and sweetened carbonated soft drinks, all of the sports drinks it analyzed had pH values low enough to cause demineralization of tooth enamel, the precursor to cavities.

COCA-COLA A SPORTS DRINK?

I will admit it: Neither my coauthor nor I could have finished this book without Coca-Cola. In our respective, predominantly healthy diets, the big red can, the sugar, and the caffeine still loom as the last temptation we indulge without regret. So you can imagine our excitement over finding this: In a 1997 survey of professional cyclists from eleven countries, all the riders on six of the eleven teams drank Coca-Cola during the last half to last quarter of the race. They drank it in addition to a carbohydrate electrolyte sports drink and, in most cases, it was flat. Riders on eight of the eleven teams also drank Coca-Cola with a sports drink after the race as well. Scientists are at a loss to explain what exactly it is about Coca-Cola that makes it so popular with these elite athletes, but they note that it's a long tradition.

The answer is yes, but the degree to which your body "loses" the benefits of exercise depends on several factors. Most important, that loss is not always as inevitable as you might think. If illness, injury, personal crisis, or other problems break your regular exercise routine, here's what you can expect to lose and how you can cut your losses.

Cardiovascular Strength

How sharply your cardiovascular fitness declines depends on the shape you were in to begin with. Physically fit people maintain their cardiovascular fitness for about twelve weeks, while people who have much lower fitness levels maintain theirs for only a few weeks before a steep decline. Interestingly, highly trained athletes show the most dramatic drop in the first weeks, but it slows after that.

Muscle Strength and Tone

As anyone who's been laid up with an injury or illness can attest, it doesn't take more than a week of inactivity to make you feel significantly weaker. Overall, however, the more fit you are, the longer it takes for inactivity to take its toll.

Athletic Performance

How much you lose depends on your level of skill and how long since you've last engaged in a sport or activity. Inactivity can lower your endurance and dull your skills, though to what degree is an individual matter. In one study, marathoners who did not train for fifteen days showed a 25 percent drop in endurance time.

What to Do to Maintain Fitness

You've worked hard to achieve a level of fitness. Don't just give it up without a fight.

- If illness or injury is interfering with your ability to exercise, ask your doctor what activities you can engage in or if you qualify for physical therapy, which can help you maintain strength. Whatever you do, take it slow and easy. Here, warmup and cool-down are especially important, and you should always stop exercising if you feel any pain, discomfort, or fatigue. Better to take a day off, rest, and try again than to risk injuring yourself or setting back your recovery. Weight training with light weights and circuit weight training (a program that combines a variety of aerobic exercises with weight training each session), gentle walking, swimming, and cycling are all good for overall fitness and keeping your bones strong.

- Consider the pool. Water running, water aerobics, aqua-cize, and swimming are generally low-impact activities that use a full range of motion. Water work can be as gentle or as challenging as you like. Of course, check with your physician first.

- If circumstances preclude following your usual workout routine (say, because you're away from home caring for a relative), find something else that you can do. Use the time to try something new. Exercise is exercise, and while walking a couple of miles on a country road isn't quite the same workout you got in your health club's high-impact step class, it's infinitely better than doing nothing. Maybe this is a good time to try yoga or dancing.

- Adjust your calorie intake to reflect your new activity level, provided you eat enough to help your body heal if you are injured or ill.

- Don't give up. Even if you lose some of your fitness edge, remember you're in a better place physically than you would have been if you hadn't taken such good care of yourself to begin with. Having reached a level of fitness before will make it easier to obtain again.

HOW TO KEEP FIT ON THE ROAD: YOUR PRIVATE HOTEL ROOM GYM

Traveling—whether for business or for pleasure—is stressful. With all the change in routine, it's easy to neglect your exercise regimen. Don't. Much of the stress, not to mention the stiff muscles that often come with getting to wherever we're going, can be alleviated with these three simple exercises. Best of all, you can find every piece of equipment you need right in your hotel room (and come to think of it, in your home too).

Power Crunch

1. Lie on your back on the floor, with your feet flat on the floor, your knees bent. Fold your arms across your chest. Raise your upper body slightly off the floor, keeping your lower back pressed against the floor.

2. Crunch your torso toward your knees, sitting up as far as you comfortably can without straining your neck muscles. Hold for two seconds, then slowly return to starting position. Do three sets of eight reps.

Chair Extension

1. Sit in a straight-back chair with your feet flat on the floor, shoulder width apart, and your hands resting on the top of your thighs.

2. With your right foot flexed, slowly extend your right leg without locking your knee over a count of two. Slowly bring your leg back to the starting position. Then raise your left leg. Repeat, alternating legs for three sets of eight reps each.

And Don't Forget Walking, Jogging, and Running

Chances are, you can walk, jog, or run almost anywhere. There's no better way to get to know a new place. Before you go out, check with the hotel's concierge, a local running club, or residents about areas in town that might not be safe or particularly amenable to walkers and runners. If for some reason running through the streets isn't possible, inquire at your hotel about fitness facilities on the premises or access to other facilities (for instance, at commercial health clubs, local schools and universities, or municipal recreation centers).

NO MORE ACHING BACK

So many adults—over 80 percent—suffer from backaches that developing a back problem seems almost inevitable. But it doesn't have to be that way. There's a lot you can do to keep your back strong and healthy, from building the best bones you can (see "Learn the B, C, D's of Better Bones," page 186) and providing optimum support with strong abdominal muscles (see "Four Minutes to Tight Abs," page 108) to learning how to slow the progress of arthritis (see "You're Never Too Young to Think About Arthritis," page 243). Ultimately, though, we have to learn to use, not abuse, our backs.

Work with Your Back, Not Against It

- **MAINTAIN A HEALTHY WEIGHT.** Extra weight puts extra strain on the back.

- **EXERCISE REGULARLY AND SENSIBLY.** And always make sure you warm up thoroughly.

- **WEAR THE RIGHT SHOES, WHATEVER YOU'RE DOING.** That means eliminate high heels or wear them only on occasion, and only for brief periods.

- **WATCH YOUR POSTURE.** Once again, Mother was right. Stand and walk tall— head high, abdominal muscles contracted, and your rib cage lifted over your hips.

- **SIT CORRECTLY.** Sit with your feet flat on the floor or on a short stool or other raised surface (such as a phone book). Do not cross your legs, since it "twists" your pelvis and your spine. When you sit, try not to "melt" back into your chair.

- **WATCH HOW YOU STAND.** Do not shift your weight from one leg to another. If you must stand for a long period of time, rest one foot on a low stool or box. When you're standing at the kitchen sink, open the cabinet door under the sink and rest your foot on the bottom shelf.

- **LEARN TO SQUAT, RATHER THAN BEND.** Stand with your feet flat on the ground, about shoulder distance apart. Slowly squat without bending at the waist. Straighten your back and then rise. Hold on to a counter or chair for support, if you must.

- **LIFT WITH SPECIAL CARE.** First and foremost, never attempt to lift anything that is too heavy for you. If you feel you can handle the weight, stand close to the object with your feet flat on the ground and shoulder distance apart, so you form a stable base of support. Squat down while keeping your back straight and bending at the knees and the hips—*not at the waist.* Think before you lift: Isolate the muscles you'll want to use—legs, buttocks, arms (also keep your abdominal muscles contracted)—then move slowly and deliberately.

- **LEARN TO MOVE IN ONE DIRECTION AT A TIME.** Become more conscious of how many directions you pull yourself in at the same time. Turning to speak to someone while reaching; rising from a chair while turning to walk in the opposite direction; and sitting up in bed, swinging your legs over the side, and standing in one seamless motion are asking for trouble. If you care for young children whom you often carry around while performing other tasks, be especially careful.

- **DON'T GET "STUCK."** Going through your daily routine with a phone receiver stuck between your ear and your hunched-up shoulder; packing a heavy shoulder bag, backpack, or diaper bag; or doing anything that stresses your muscles is likely to prompt them to rebel, and muscles in revolt often go on strike. That's called a spasm. Whatever you're doing, break the position, move around, and give your back a break.

- **GIVE YOUR BACK A GOOD NIGHT'S REST.** The best position for sleeping is on either side with your legs drawn up a bit. Lying on your back is fine, if you like it, as long as your knees and neck are supported. Sleeping on your stomach should be avoided, if you can. Find a pillow that supports your cervical (neck) spine so that it remains relatively straight. Very soft pillows can let the cervical vertebrae "curve."

If You Experience Chronic, Severe, or Debilitating Back Pain

It's time to seek medical attention if:

- your back pain is severe, chronic, or debilitating;

- you experience numbness, shooting pains, or a loss of function anywhere in your body (for example, a weakened grip or loss of bladder control);

- your back pain doesn't seem to improve with your usual home-treatment regimen (over-the-counter pain relievers, heat, and rest).

There are many causes of back pain, from simple muscle strain to degeneration of the spine, that can result in disability or paralysis. Only a physician, preferably an orthopedist or a doctor of chiropractic medicine, can accurately diagnose your particular problem.

Remember: The pain of muscles in spasm is really your body's way of protecting your back. By "freezing" muscles in place, your body prevents movement that could result in further injury. Regard pain as a warning sign, not as an enemy. Before you embark on a regimen of painkillers and muscle relaxants, be sure you understand the real cause of your problem. Symptom relief alone is fine for the short term, but your goal should be to discover and do all you can to avoid future problems through physical therapy and the right exercise program.

SELF-MASSAGE TIPS FOR THAT ACHING LOWER BACK

Deep pressure stimulates blood flow, which can help muscles relax and hasten healing.

1. With your fingers pointing downward, firmly stroke along the lower spine, fanning your hands over your hips, then sliding your hands back up. Repeat this six times.

2. With your hands resting on your hips, apply pressure along your spine with your thumbs. Release and repeat an inch higher, continuing up as far as you can reach comfortably.

3. Lie on your back on a firm surface, such as the floor. Bend your knees so that your feet are flat on the floor. Tilt your pelvis slightly so that the natural curve of

your back is flattened, and you can feel your lower vertebrae against the floor. Bend your knees, slowly drawing them to your chest, then hold them there gently for thirty seconds or a minute. Release and relax.

GETTING THROUGH THE TRANSITION

No matter how great your workouts are going or how successful your new approach to eating, one day you'll wake up and think to yourself, "Is this it?" When that happens, you've hit the transition, the point where you're closing in on or have reached your original goals and need a new horizon to shoot for. Many people get lost in the transition because they attribute their new ambivalence to "boredom." But it's much more than that. And when you recognize and plan for this tricky passage, you'll be able to come through it stronger and more committed than before.

Sometimes the way through it is obvious. You might try making your workout more challenging or getting more exercise outside the gym—say, by taking up hiking. Or you might decide to push forward with a long-range plan to eat an even healthier diet. Sometimes those kinds of solutions work. But it's important to remember that anything you do for your body isn't just about your body. It's about you. Once you recognize that, it's easy to see what change might spark your enthusiasm and keep you going.

When you hit that slump, look beyond what you're doing about diet and exercise to find new answers. Bear in mind that for many people, the transition comes when their minds haven't quite caught up to the other changes they've made.

You know you've hit the transition when:

- you begin finding good, valid excuses for missing workouts;

- you don't get the same satisfaction out of reaching your goals that you did before;

- you begin taking your accomplishments for granted.

You can survive the transition and come out better for it by:

- talking to someone who knows you and understands your attitude toward fitness, preferably someone who's witnessed the changes you've gone through;

- setting new goals you find exciting;

- trying new activities, making it a point to learn more about exercise or nutrition, or taking classes with a new teacher.

Record Your Goals

Before you begin making any major changes in your health—no matter how minor or grand—always write down in a small notebook why you're doing it. You don't have to write a book, but you should spend at least fifteen minutes putting down on paper what you feel about yourself and why these changes are important to you. Write about what you hope to accomplish and what it means to you. Keep this by your bed and look at it as often as you need to, to remind yourself why you started and what you want to achieve.

grain, pasta, or rice is also about the size of your fist; double that for main-dish servings

...E WHAT YOU CONSIDER "PROBLEM FOODS" IN SINGLE-SERVE ...S. Although it costs a little more to purchase foods in individually ... or single-serving packages, until you feel you have a realistic and fairly ... idea of what constitutes a serving, it may well be worth your while. For ..., rather than buy the whole pint of chocolate sorbet or a big chunk of ... purchase chocolate sorbet pops and individually wrapped cheese slices. ...emima frozen pancakes, for example, come packed with exactly three ...kes—one portion—per pouch; gelatin, yogurt, applesauce, canned fruit, ice ..., cottage cheese, and puddings all come individually packaged in "snack"

...GH AND MEASURE EVERYTHING FOR A WEEK. This eye opener is well ...th the effort. I assure you, you'll never look at a heaping plate of pasta or a ...ounce steak the same way again.

...YOU FAIL TO CONTROL YOUR PORTION, IT DOESN'T MEAN YOU HAVE TO ...OSE CONTROL OF YOUR DIET. Be honest with yourself. If you ate five cookies ...nstead of three, three servings of soup instead of just one, note the difference in ...calories and compensate for it over the next day or so. Remember, it's not eating ...too much of any one food that's the problem—it's eating more calories than you ...expend over the course of several days or more. Two extra cookies may mean no ...salad dressing with dinner; that extra soup, no low-fat hot cocoa before bed or no ...peanut butter with tomorrow morning's English muffin.

CHOOSE AND LOSE

No one can diet forever. Long-term weight-loss success is based on learning how to eat better while enjoying yourself. There's no need to fill your grocery cart with the high-priced, fake-fat, artificially sweetened stuff the diet-food industry tries to pass off as satisfying and good for you. Getting through your weight-loss program with fake-food rewards is like trying to win the Tour de France with training wheels on: It's not

Getting the Most from the Foods You Eat

4.

. . . .

Like so many people I've worked with, Susan was a veteran of the Diet Wars. Eager and willing to devote her energy to doing whatever would make her look better, Susan was easily swept up by one food philosophy or another. First it was a low-fat regimen that left her with thinning hair, constant skin problems, intense PMS, and a perpetual cold. After a series of binges, Susan concluded that this plan wasn't for her.

She was tired of feeling tired, so she gravitated toward a super-high-protein plan that had her eating at least twice the amount of protein her body could use. Once her enthusiasm over her new "foodstyle" change wore off, she began feeling a little bit worn her-self. Her skin was still dry, she felt weak, and her boyfriend even commented on how often she was using the restroom. She was losing weight, but—although she didn't know it—most of it was muscle mass, not body fat. Every time she urinated, precious calcium and magnesium were being washed away, another side effect of the body trying to metabolize too much protein.

Feeling drained, Susan decided to try something a coworker raved about, a high-carbohydrate, low-calorie diet. The bulk of her daily menu consisted of grains, pastas, fruits, and vegetables, with a small amount of protein. Susan, who loved carbohydrate foods, took to this plan right away. But before long, she began having intense cravings and feeling as if she just didn't have the energy to make it through the day. In an effort to distract herself from the binge that was looming like a Thanksgiving Day–parade balloon, Susan became a connoisseur of low-fat, no-fat, artificially sweetened, fake-fat "treats" that were never satisfying and left a strange aftertaste.

"I've tried everything, but nothing works," she lamented the first time we sat down to talk. After she had a thorough physical checkup with her doctor, who also ordered an intensive series of blood tests, what I suspected was confirmed: Susan was losing muscle tone, not consuming enough calories, and not getting enough exercise. Working with her over several months, we changed all that with a balanced diet that included the right proportions of protein, carbohydrates, and fat. The results were incredible, and everything you need to know to strike that perfect balance is right here.

SERVE YOURSELF RIGHT: SIZE UP A SERVING

I've said this already but I can't emphasize i[...] we are accustomed to eating. All information [...] of a food is based on a specific, stated portion [...] what most of us already suspect: We eat more—[...] more of everything else—than what the Nutri[...] "serving size." Most of us underestimate our daily [...]

Weight-reduction experts often speak of "po[...] jumping out of the package, crowding its way onto [...] What we're really talking about here is "consumer c[...] then eat the correct portions.

- **READ AND FOLLOW THE LABEL.** While it's not alw[...] serving size, making a point of doing so for a few we[...] much is enough. Always read how many servings are [...] it's two or more, divide the food or beverage according[...] pretzels contains two servings, pour half out into a bow[...] and put it away. If a "serving" is three cookies, take out t[...] package, and put it away before you take the first bite. Do[...] open package and trust yourself to stop once you've eaten [...]

- **DON'T MUNCH WHILE YOU'RE COOKING OR PREPARING F**[...] Swiss cheese you ate while making the sandwiches for lunch c[...] the couple of tablespoons of "leftover" frosting, probably anoth[...] must taste, make it a rule to taste only what you could fit in a sc[...]

- **LEARN WHAT A PORTION LOOKS LIKE.**

  3 ounces cooked meat or chicken (4 ounces uncooked) is about 3 by [...] inches, about the size of the palm of your hand
  4 ounces fish (5 ounces uncooked) is a little bit larger, depending on i[...] thickness
  a medium piece of fruit is approximately the same size as your fist with y[...] thumb held up; a medium banana measures about 5 inches long

½ cup of a[...] quantity [...]

- PURCHA[...]
  PACKAG[...]
  wrapped [...]
  accurat[...]
  exampl[...]
  cheese[...]
  Aunt J[...]
  panca[...]
  crean[...]
  sizes[...]

- WE[...]
  wo[...]
  12[...]

- IF[...]
  L[...]

Getting the Most from the Foods You Eat

4.

Like so many people I've worked with, Susan was a veteran of the Diet Wars. Eager and willing to devote her energy to doing whatever would make her look better, Susan was easily swept up by one food philosophy or another. First it was a low-fat regimen that left her with thinning hair, constant skin problems, intense PMS, and a perpetual cold. After a series of binges, Susan concluded that this plan wasn't for her.

She was tired of feeling tired, so she gravitated toward a super-high-protein plan that had her eating at least twice the amount of protein her body could use. Once her enthusiasm over her new "foodstyle" change wore off, she began feeling a little bit worn herself. Her skin was still dry, she felt weak, and her boyfriend even commented on how often she was using the restroom. She was losing weight, but—although she didn't know it—most of it was muscle mass, not body fat. Every time she urinated, precious calcium and magnesium were being washed away, another side effect of the body trying to metabolize too much protein.

Feeling drained, Susan decided to try something a coworker raved about, a high-carbohydrate, low-calorie diet. The bulk of her daily menu consisted of grains, pastas, fruits, and vegetables, with a small amount of protein. Susan, who loved carbohydrate foods, took to this plan right away. But before long, she began having intense cravings and feeling as if she just didn't have the energy to make it through the day. In an effort to distract herself from the binge that was looming like a Thanksgiving Day–parade balloon, Susan became a connoisseur of low-fat, no-fat, artificially sweetened, fake-fat "treats" that were never satisfying and left a strange aftertaste.

"I've tried everything, but nothing works," she lamented the first time we sat down to talk. After she had a thorough physical checkup with her doctor, who also ordered an intensive series of blood tests, what I suspected was confirmed: Susan was losing muscle tone, not consuming enough calories, and not getting enough exercise. Working with her over several months, we changed all that with a balanced diet that included the right proportions of protein, carbohydrates, and fat. The results were incredible, and everything you need to know to strike that perfect balance is right here.

SERVE YOURSELF RIGHT: LEARN TO SIZE UP A SERVING

I've said this already but I can't emphasize it enough: A serving is not however much we are accustomed to eating. All information on the composition and calorie content of a food is based on a specific, stated portion size. Numerous studies have confirmed what most of us already suspect: We eat more—and get more calories, more fat, and more of everything else—than what the Nutrition Facts outline as an appropriate "serving size." Most of us underestimate our daily caloric intake by 20 to 40 percent!

Weight-reduction experts often speak of "portion control" as if the food were jumping out of the package, crowding its way onto the plate like a rampaging mob. What we're really talking about here is "consumer control"—learning to identify and then eat the correct portions.

- **READ AND FOLLOW THE LABEL.** While it's not always easy to stick to the serving size, making a point of doing so for a few weeks will help you learn how much is enough. Always read how many servings are contained in the product. If it's two or more, divide the food or beverage accordingly. For example, if a bag of pretzels contains two servings, pour half out into a bowl, then reseal the package and put it away. If a "serving" is three cookies, take out three cookies, close the package, and put it away before you take the first bite. Don't sit there with an open package and trust yourself to stop once you've eaten your portion.

- **DON'T MUNCH WHILE YOU'RE COOKING OR PREPARING FOOD.** That slice of Swiss cheese you ate while making the sandwiches for lunch cost 100 calories, the couple of tablespoons of "leftover" frosting, probably another 100. If you must taste, make it a rule to taste only what you could fit in a scant teaspoon.

- **LEARN WHAT A PORTION LOOKS LIKE.**

  3 ounces cooked meat or chicken (4 ounces uncooked) is about 3 by 5 inches, about the size of the palm of your hand
  4 ounces fish (5 ounces uncooked) is a little bit larger, depending on its thickness
  a medium piece of fruit is approximately the same size as your fist with your thumb held up; a medium banana measures about 5 inches long

½ cup of a grain, pasta, or rice is also about the size of your fist; double that
  quantity for main-dish servings

- **PURCHASE WHAT YOU CONSIDER "PROBLEM FOODS" IN SINGLE-SERVE
  PACKAGES.** Although it costs a little more to purchase foods in individually
  wrapped or single-serving packages, until you feel you have a realistic and fairly
  accurate idea of what constitutes a serving, it may well be worth your while. For
  example, rather than buy the whole pint of chocolate sorbet or a big chunk of
  cheese, purchase chocolate sorbet pops and individually wrapped cheese slices.
  Aunt Jemima frozen pancakes, for example, come packed with exactly three
  pancakes—one portion—per pouch; gelatin, yogurt, applesauce, canned fruit, ice
  cream, cottage cheese, and puddings all come individually packaged in "snack"
  sizes.

- **WEIGH AND MEASURE EVERYTHING FOR A WEEK.** This eye opener is well
  worth the effort. I assure you, you'll never look at a heaping plate of pasta or a
  12-ounce steak the same way again.

- **IF YOU FAIL TO CONTROL YOUR PORTION, IT DOESN'T MEAN YOU HAVE TO
  LOSE CONTROL OF YOUR DIET.** Be honest with yourself. If you ate five cookies
  instead of three, three servings of soup instead of just one, note the difference in
  calories and compensate for it over the next day or so. Remember, it's not eating
  too much of any one food that's the problem—it's eating more calories than you
  expend over the course of several days or more. Two extra cookies may mean no
  salad dressing with dinner; that extra soup, no low-fat hot cocoa before bed or no
  peanut butter with tomorrow morning's English muffin.

CHOOSE AND LOSE

No one can diet forever. Long-term weight-loss success is based on learning how
to eat better while enjoying yourself. There's no need to fill your grocery cart with the
high-priced, fake-fat, artificially sweetened stuff the diet-food industry tries to pass off
as satisfying and good for you. Getting through your weight-loss program with fake-
food rewards is like trying to win the Tour de France with training wheels on: It's not

pleasurable, rewarding, fulfilling, or even fun. And you know, those wheels have to come off someday. Start now developing the habits you'll want to keep for a lifetime, and never worry about your weight again.

CHOOSE . . .	INSTEAD OF . . .
chocolate sorbet bar	chocolate-covered ice cream bar
broiled chicken sandwich without skin	fried chicken sandwich
plain popcorn, air-popped, 1 cup	peanuts, raw, ½ cup
pasta with marinara sauce, 1 cup	pasta with meat sauce, 1 cup
steamed clams, 1 cup	fried clams, 1 cup
plain low-fat yogurt, 1 cup	sour cream, 1 cup
part-skim cheese, 2 oz.	whole milk cheese, 2 oz.
tuna in water	tuna in oil
baked apple, unsweetened	apple pie, 1 slice
salsa, ½ cup	guacamole, ½ cup
iced cappuccino with skim milk, 12 oz.	chocolate milk shake, 12 oz.
unsweetened shredded wheat, ½ cup	granola with raisins and dates, ½ cup
flavored seltzer, 1 glass	soft drink, 1 glass
egg-white omelette, 3 eggs	whole-egg omelette, 3 eggs
veggie burger patty	beef hamburger patty

CHOOSE . . .	INSTEAD OF . . .
Tootsie Pop	*chocolate candy bar*
angel food cake, no frosting	*jelly donut*
broth, 1 cup	*cream soup, 1 cup*
light beer, 12 oz.	*premium beer, 12 oz.*
skim milk, 1 cup	*whole milk, 1 cup*
fresh apricots, 2	*dried apricots, ½ cup*
fresh pear, 1	*canned pears, 2 halves in heavy syrup*

POTATO: BAKED VS. FRIED—A BIG DIFFERENCE

| | | | FAT, IN GRAMS | |
	CALORIES	SATURATED	MONOUNSATURATED	POLYUNSATURATED
1 potato, baked with skin, no salt, 5½ oz.	164	0.039	0.003	0.065
1 potato, french fried in vegetable oil, 5½ oz.	457	3.840	9.870	5.500

PROTEIN: PRO AND CON

Everywhere you turn, it seems somebody's pushing protein, and so it has always been. Growing up, we learned to place protein on a nutritional pedestal and to value protein foods—overwhelmingly those from animal sources, such as meat, eggs, fish, and dairy products—as the healthiest. The same thinking governs the perennially popular hype surrounding high-protein weight-loss diets and high-protein dietary supplements. If you didn't know any better, you'd think we were all suffering from a protein shortage. In fact, most of us get too much protein every day, and this excess has a definite, negative impact on health.

Pro Protein

Protein is essential to health. Our hormones, genes, enzymes, antibodies, hair, skin, muscles, bones, blood, cartilage, and major organs consist of some percentage of protein. Our bodies break down the protein we consume into amino acids, the so-called building blocks of our physical beings. There are twenty-two amino acids, and our bodies can create all but nine of these. The nine we must consume are called essential amino acids, and one reason animal products have been viewed as "superior" protein sources is that they usually contain the nine essential amino acids, among others. The protein we derive from vegetable sources is called "incomplete" because it contains a limited number of amino acids, and usually small quantities of the nine essential amino acids. However, you can get enough protein without eating animal products by being sure that over the course of a day, you get all the essential amino acids from what you do eat. (See page 137.)

It's important to eat the protein you need every day, because the body does not store excess protein the way it stores calories from fat or carbohydrates, and here's where some people get confused. Just because your body cannot store protein as protein doesn't mean that any calories you get from eating protein can't be turned to fat. They can. Every gram of protein contains 4 calories. While your body cannot store amino acids for future use, it does hang on to those calories and "shelves" them as body fat.

Protein requirements are based on body weight and activity level. Currently the Recommended Daily Allowance (RDA) is 50 grams for adults. (RDAs for pregnant women, nursing mothers, and children are different.) If you want to determine your protein requirements more specifically, convert your weight in pounds to kilograms:

your weight $\times$ 0.45 = _____ kilograms

Then multiply your weight in kilograms by one of the following numbers:

0.6 for sedentary to moderately active

1.1 for active

1.2 for strength athletes

1.5 for athletes who train for endurance and for strength

1.7 for endurance athletes

How much protein do you have to eat to meet those requirements? Probably a lot less than you think. For example, a 3-ounce serving of beef, chicken, or fish—which is about the size of a deck of playing cards—supplies 21 grams of protein, about 40 percent of the RDA. On average, protein should not make up more than 10 to 15 percent of your calorie intake for a day. So, for example, if you eat 1,800 calories a day, you would multiply that number by 10 to 15 percent to find out how many of those calories should be protein (180–270). Then divide that by 4 (since there are 4 calories per gram of protein) to determine how many grams of protein it will take to achieve your required protein calories (in this example, 45–67.5). (See charts.)

PROTEIN REQUIREMENTS (IN GRAMS) FOR YOUR WEIGHT AND ACTIVITY LEVEL

BODY WEIGHT		ACTIVITY LEVEL					
POUNDS	KILOGRAMS	SEDENTARY (× 0.6)	MODERATE (× 0.8)	ACTIVE (× 1.1)	STRENGTH (× 1.2)	COMBINATION (× 1.5)	ENDURANCE (× 1.7)
90	40.5	24.3	32.4	44.6	48.6	60.8	68.9
95	42.8	25.7	34.2	47.0	51.3	64.1	72.7
100	45.0	27.0	36.0	49.5	54.0	67.5	76.5
105	47.3	28.4	37.8	52.0	56.7	70.9	80.3
110	49.5	29.7	39.6	54.5	59.4	74.3	84.2
115	51.8	31.1	41.4	56.9	62.1	77.6	88.0
120	54.0	32.4	43.2	59.4	64.8	81.0	91.8
125	56.3	33.8	45.0	61.9	67.5	84.4	95.6
130	58.5	35.1	46.8	64.4	70.2	87.8	99.5
135	60.8	36.5	48.6	66.8	72.9	91.1	103.3
140	63.0	37.8	50.4	69.3	75.6	94.5	107.1
145	65.3	39.2	52.2	71.8	78.3	97.9	110.9
150	67.5	40.5	54.0	74.3	81.0	101.3	114.8
155	69.8	41.9	55.8	76.7	83.7	104.6	118.6
160	72.0	43.2	57.6	79.2	86.4	108.0	122.4
165	74.3	44.6	59.4	81.7	89.1	111.4	126.2
170	76.5	45.9	61.2	84.2	91.8	114.8	130.1
175	78.8	47.3	63.0	86.6	94.5	118.1	133.9
180	81.0	48.6	64.8	89.1	97.2	121.5	137.7
185	83.3	50.0	66.6	91.6	99.9	124.9	141.5
190	85.5	51.3	68.4	94.1	102.6	128.3	145.4
195	87.8	52.7	70.2	96.5	105.3	131.6	149.2
200	90.0	54.0	72.0	99.0	108.0	135.0	153.0

Note: Figures rounded off to nearest tenth.

PROTEIN REQUIREMENTS (IN GRAMS) FOR YOUR WEIGHT AND ACTIVITY LEVEL (continued)

BODY WEIGHT		ACTIVITY LEVEL					
POUNDS	KILOGRAMS	SEDENTARY (× 0.6)	MODERATE (× 0.8)	ACTIVE (× 1.1)	STRENGTH (× 1.2)	COMBINATION (× 1.5)	ENDURANCE (× 1.7)
205	92.3	55.4	73.8	101.5	110.7	138.4	156.8
210	94.5	56.7	75.6	104.0	113.4	141.8	160.7
215	96.8	58.1	77.4	106.4	116.1	145.1	164.5
220	99.0	59.4	79.2	108.9	118.8	148.5	168.3
225	101.3	60.8	81.0	111.4	121.5	151.9	172.1
230	103.5	62.1	82.8	113.9	124.2	155.3	176.0
235	105.8	63.5	84.6	116.3	126.9	158.6	179.8

Note: Figures rounded off to nearest tenth.

RECOMMENDED DAILY PROTEIN (GR.)

total daily calories	10% protein	15% protein
1,000	25	37.5
1,200	30	45
1,400	35	52.5
1,600	40	60
1,800	45	67.5
2,000	50	75
2,200	55	82.5
2,400	60	90
2,600	65	97.5
2,800	70	105
3,000	75	112.5

You may need more protein if you are pregnant, nursing, or seriously or chronically ill. Consult your doctor or a nutritionist.

What's Wrong with Protein?

Contrary to popular belief, athletes don't need more protein because they need more energy but because they're constantly repairing and building muscle tissue. In fact, protein is a relatively poor source of energy, so don't waste your money on "protein" candy bars or high-protein drinks and shakes because you think they'll "supercharge" your workout. And there's no scientific proof that protein or amino acid supplements build more muscle faster. In fact, some experts point out that we're really not sure yet that amino acid supplements are safe over the long term.

When we talk about what's "wrong" with protein, the problem is not protein itself but the demands we place on our bodies when called to metabolize more than we need. Here's what you risk when your protein intake exceeds your needs.

- **DEHYDRATION.** Your body uses more water to metabolize protein than it does to metabolize either carbohydrates or fats.

- **CALCIUM DEFICIENCY AND, EVENTUALLY, OSTEOPOROSIS.** A Japanese study found that people who ate 5 ounces or more of meat (beef or chicken) daily excreted significantly more calcium in their urine than vegetarians. In recent years, there have been some conflicting studies that suggest the protein–calcium-loss connection is not so clear.

- **MUSCLE FATIGUE.** In the simplest terms, your muscles require glycogen, which is best derived from carbohydrates. Eating too much protein and not enough carbohydrates makes it difficult for your body to replace the glycogen expended during your workouts, resulting in fatigue.

- **COMPROMISED KIDNEY FUNCTION, AND EVENTUALLY KIDNEY DISEASE.** When you metabolize protein, it gets split three ways: (1) the amino acids that your body will use for growth, repair, and maintenance of tissues and fluids; (2) calories that your body will use for energy or store as fat; and (3) excess nitrogen from the amino acids, which passes through the liver, where it is converted to urea before going on to the kidneys for excretion. From the kidneys' point of view, protein molecules are large and difficult to process. Healthy kidneys can handle this burden with ease, but millions of us have diminished kidney function and don't even know it. That's because renal function can be reduced by 90 percent or more before symptoms appear. Also, kidney function tends to decline naturally with age.

- **THE OTHER ISSUES "TRADITIONAL" PROTEINS RAISE.** Meats, fish, eggs, and dairy products can be high in saturated fat and contain hormones, antibiotics, and pesticides of questionable long-term safety. Gram for gram, protein from animal sources (with the exception of eggs) is generally more expensive than that from plant sources. And the recent surge in the number of bacterial food-poisoning incidents is yet another reason to reconsider our overreliance on these "traditional" protein sources. Decades of studies point to links between high protein consumption and heart disease and some cancers (breast, prostate, uterus, pancreas, kidney, rectum, and colon). Whether the culprit is the actual protein itself, its aforementioned "traveling" companions (fat, pesticides, preservatives, etc.), or the by-product of its metabolism is unclear.

- **DETHRONE KING PROTEIN.** Commit to memory a new protein mantra: *Too much of a good thing is a bad thing.*

- **EAT ONLY THE PROTEIN YOU NEED.** See the chart on page 133 to determine how many grams of protein you need.

- **STRIKE THE RIGHT BALANCE.** If you haven't done it already, try to derive at least two-thirds (or more) of your protein from plant sources, such as soybean products, nuts, seeds, legumes and beans, cereals, and grains. These sources all offer other benefits, including lower fat, virtually no hormone or antibiotic residues, and a range of nutritional pluses (fiber, vitamins, minerals, monounsaturated or polyunsaturated fat, etc.). Take a few minutes to learn about the food combinations that result in complete proteins (see below). You'll be surprised at how many you eat already.

- **DON'T FALL FOR THE HYPE.** If you feel tired after your workout, you probably need more carbohydrates, not more protein. If your friend has dropped several pounds on a high-protein diet, remember the golden rule of fad-dieting success: Any diet that severely restricts food choice will result in temporary weight loss. If your nails are cracking and your ends are splitting—yet you're eating enough protein—look to changes in your diet overall and your lifestyle before you plunk down money for protein or amino-acid supplements.

Complete Protein without Meat

The following combinations of incomplete protein foods result in dishes whose complete protein value meets or exceeds that of meat and animal products. Also remember, these foods need not be in the same dish, just in the same meal. For example, you might create your complete protein for lunch by adding chickpeas to your salad and rice to your casserole. If you're concerned about cholesterol and dietary fat, most of an egg's amino acids are in the fat-free white. (See "The Good Egg," page 138.)

WITH . . .	ADD . . .
rice	black beans
pasta	cheese
legumes: black-eyed peas, chickpeas, kidney beans, lentils, lima beans, navy beans, peanuts, pinto beans, soybeans, split (but not fresh) peas	barley, corn, rice, sesame seeds, or wheat
tofu	rice
cereal	milk
rice	milk
peanut butter	bread

Don't Forget Vegetable Protein

We generally don't think of vegetables and grains as protein foods. Though they aren't as protein-dense as animal flesh and products, if you're eating all the servings you need, you may be getting more protein (though incomplete) than you realize. A medium baked potato, a cup of broccoli, and half a cup of green peas contain about 4 grams each of protein. A cup of egg noodles, macaroni, or spaghetti each has about 6 grams.

THE GOOD EGG

Once upon a time, the egg was the star of the all-American breakfast. Along with bacon, buttered toast, whole milk, and maybe even a side of pancakes, the egg sent millions of us out to face the day with a full quota of carbohydrates and protein, along with a nice serving of saturated fat and cholesterol. Everyone loved the egg until the 1970s, when studies emerged associating high dietary fat intake with coronary artery disease.

These studies fingered a range of high-fat and high-cholesterol foods, including our sunny little friend, as culprits in our rising levels of heart disease. The egg, it later turned out, wasn't so bad after all.

The egg was guilty by association (it was the saturated fat and cholesterol in the accompanying bacon and butter that did most of the damage). While it's true that eggs are loaded with both cholesterol (213 milligrams each, all in the yolk) and saturated fat (5 grams), only one of these fat grams is the type of saturated fat that clogs arteries. Despite the egg's high cholesterol count, its effect on most people's blood cholesterol level is an insignificant 3 milligrams. That's why the American Heart Association has revised its recommendations to allow four egg yolks per week. And in early 1999, a long-term study of over 117,000 people found that, for most, those who ate an egg a day had no greater health risks than those who ate just one a week.

More good news is that the egg is one of nature's near-perfect foods. It's inexpensive and easy to prepare in a number of ways. One hard-boiled or poached egg provides 6 grams of protein along with substantial percentages of your RDAs for iron, zinc, phosphorus, vitamins A, D, B_3, B_{12}, and pantothenic acid. Obviously, how "good" the egg is depends a lot on how you prepare it.

- Hard-boiled, poached, or cooked in a nonstick pan without additional oil are the best ways.

- Don't overlook the "pure protein/no fat" values of egg whites alone, prepared as an omelette or a salad for sandwiches (for example, low-fat salad dressing with chopped egg whites, spices, and cooked, drained and chopped spinach).

- To reduce cholesterol in your egg dishes, remove the yolks of half or more eggs (for example, make French toast with two whole eggs and three whites).

GOT MILK?

We all grew up believing that milk and dairy products were the essence of wholesome, healthy goodness. Dairy products are rich in calcium, protein, and, in low- and no-fat versions, are a great "calorie bargain." Most dairy foods have a satisfying consistency, and our childhood associations to foods liked grilled cheese sandwiches, chocolate milk, ice cream, and yogurt make them irresistible comfort foods. For most of us, it's a rare meal that doesn't include some dairy product, even if it's just a pat of butter.

There are others, however, who feel that milk isn't all it's cracked up to be (see below). Yes, it is possible to live without dairy products. You can use soy or rice milk for cooking, to lighten coffee, and on your dry breakfast cereal. Soy cheeses, yogurt, and butter are becoming more widely available. But learning to meet your daily calcium requirements through diet alone takes some forethought and planning (see "Learn the B, C, D's of Better Bones," page 186).

What's Wrong with Milk?

It depends on whom you ask. Most commercially available milk and dairy products do contain traces of the antibiotics and hormones modern dairies depend on to keep the milk flowing. Whether these pose a clear danger to human health remains a matter of controversy. What is known is that many people are allergic to dairy products; it is one of the top five food allergens. Others may be sensitive to the antibiotics and hormones milk contains or be unable to digest lactose—the sugar in milk—properly. Recent research suggests that one in three people who believe they are lactose-intolerant actually can drink up to two glasses of milk a day without any ill effect, as long as several hours pass between the first glass and the second.

Some people find that forgoing dairy products makes them feel better in general. If you suffer from PMS, chronic fatigue, arthritis, asthma, chronic allergies, or lactose intolerance (gas, cramps, and diarrhea after eating dairy foods), you might try abstaining for a few weeks and see how you feel. Or switch to lactose-reduced products or take lactase enzyme tablets when you do eat dairy foods. These are available under such brand names as Lactaid and Dairy Ease, as well as generic brands.

Don't overlook the possibility that the source of your problem is not the milk product itself but what you're eating with it. For instance, maybe it's not the milk in your coffee that's upsetting your stomach, but the caffeine or the high fat content of the cottage cheese you ate along with it. Or try organically produced milk that's free of antibiotics and hormones. Just be sure that it is pasteurized, not "raw," milk.

Milk Myths

- **FALSE: DAIRY FOODS INCREASE MUCUS, WHICH EXACERBATES COLDS, FLUS, AND SINUS INFECTIONS, BECAUSE GERMS AND VIRUSES FEED ON MUCUS.**

Milk does not create mucus, and viruses and bacteria do not "feed on" mucus. What dairy products do is inhibit the body's natural tendency to respond to congestion with a rush of fluid that thins mucus, so we feel less congested.

- **FALSE: IF YOU SUFFER FROM ACID INDIGESTION, DRINK MILK BECAUSE IT "COATS" THE STOMACH.** If anything, drinking milk can prompt more acid production.

- **FALSE: THERE'S NO POINT IN SWITCHING TO LOW-FAT OR SKIM MILK, SINCE WHOLE MILK IS ONLY ABOUT 3 PERCENT FAT.** Each cup of whole milk contains 8.5 grams of fat, 65 percent of which is in the form of saturated fat. Low-fat milk has 4.2 grams of fat—nearly half—and skim milk has none. If you eat 2,000 calories a day and keep your fat intake to 25 percent, two glasses of whole milk would "use up" about a quarter of your daily fat allowance.

- **FALSE: TO AVOID PESTICIDES, HORMONES, AND ANTIBIOTICS, GO FOR RAW MILK. IT'S MORE "NATURAL."** When it comes to dairy foods, "raw" does not mean "fresh" or "organic." It means that the product has not been pasteurized to kill potentially deadly bacteria that thrive in milk. Pasteurization does not destroy the nutrients in milk, so there's no reason to get it raw. In 1985 raw milk contaminated by listeria was the cause of forty-seven deaths—one of the biggest food poisoning episodes in this country. In the late 1990s public health experts cited listeria-contaminated food as a growing threat to food safety generally. *Never buy raw, unpasteurized milk or dairy products!*

FAT: UNLOCKING THE RIGHT COMBINATION

You're tracking your daily fat intake and eating the low- or no-fat versions of your favorite foods. Years ago, you tossed out butter in favor of margarine, then eliminated every trace of oil from your pantry "because they're all fattening." Out went the potato chips, in came snack crackers. If you're like most Americans, however, these changes have made virtually no difference in your weight (if anything, you've probably put on a few more pounds), and even if you've maintained a healthy weight, your doctor may have warned you that your general cholesterol and low-density cholesterol (LDL, the "bad" type) are higher than ever. What gives?

If you're confused about fat, you're in good company. Even the experts admit being puzzled by some developments that seem to defy the "Laws of Fat" as we know them:

- Why, despite eating fewer calories in fat (though that's debatable), are we still suffering the effects of fat in terms of added weight gain and high blood-cholesterol levels?

- Why do cultures where people consume up to 40 percent (a full third more than the U.S. recommendation) of daily calories in fat have *less* heart disease and other fat-related diseases than we do?

- Why do people who eat an extremely low fat (18-percent) diet still have trouble losing weight?

It seems that the type of fat may be even more important to your health than the amount. Basically, there are four types of fat: monounsaturated fats, polyunsaturated fats, saturated fats, and trans fat. If you have trouble remembering which type you should eat and in what proportions, think of it alphabetically. The highest proportion of fat calories should be derived from monounsaturated fats, followed in decreasing proportions by polyunsaturated fats, then saturated fats, and—last and least—trans fatty acids.

What Are EFAs?

We've heard of EFAs, or essential fatty acids. But what are they? Omega-3 and omega-6 fatty acids are essential to human health because they contain linolenic and linoleic acids, respectively, that our bodies need but cannot produce. To date, there are no clear guidelines on how much of each we need, but new findings suggest that they may be even more important than we think. The key is not to simply consume more omega-3 and omega-6 oils, but to do so in the correct proportion. You should strive to balance omega-3 and omega-6 oils 2:1, then eventually work up to a ratio of 1:1. Omega-3 has been shown to lower the risk of heart disease, alleviate arthritis pain, make blood less likely to clot, and enhance nervous-system function. Omega-6 fatty acids are the bio-chemical building blocks of the brain and the retina. Because omega-6 is found in common oils, such as corn, soybean, sunflower, and safflower, most of us get more than enough. Omega-3, however, is not as plentiful in most daily diets. Virtually all fish contains some omega-3, but fatty fish, such as salmon, herring, mackerel, and sardines, contains higher concentrations. You can also find it in soy products such as tofu, nuts, flaxseed and flaxseed oil, and green leafy vegetables.

The charts below outline the recommended proportions of each type of fat and its sources. As you rework the fat combinations in your diet, keep these tips in mind:

- Daily dietary fat intake should not exceed 30 percent of daily calories, no matter how "good" the fat.

- If you increase consumption of one type of fat (say, eating more monounsaturated fat, such as olive oil), be sure you reduce consumption of the others. Remember, even "good" fats contain the same number of total calories as the "bad" ones, such as lard.

- Don't fool yourself into thinking that just because you had the low-fat ice cream instead of the super-premium high-fat real thing, you can splurge on something else or go for seconds.

- "Low-" and "reduced-" fat foods still contain calories, and calories still do count. Three thousand calories of lard and 3,000 calories of fat-free sorbet or "reduced-fat" cheesecake will result in the same pound of body fat.

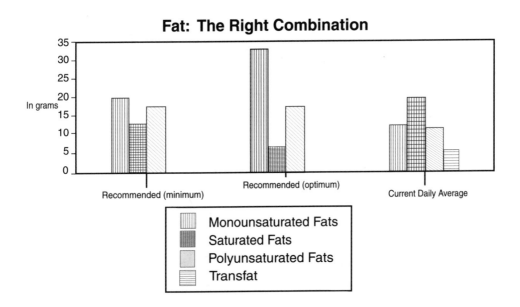

Fat: The Right Combination

FAT AT A GLANCE

Type of Fat	U.S. Department of Agriculture Recommendations		Why Eat More	Why Eat Less	Sources
	1,500 Cal./Day Diet	2,000 Cal./Day Diet			
Monounsaturated Current average is low: 12–13% of daily calories.	20–33 gr. 12–20% of total calories	27–44 gr. 12–20% of total calories	Promotes lower blood cholesterol; may protect against breast cancer.		olive oil, canola oil, peanuts and peanut oil, sunflower oil
Omega-6 fats Current average: too high a proportion of omega-6 fats in relation to omega-3.	Ideally, you should eat omega-3s and omega-6s at a ratio of 2:1, then when your body is used to it, 1:1, with more omega-3s, fewer omega-6s than you're probably eating now.		Contains linoleic acid, an essential fatty acid, which cannot be produced by the body; lowers total blood cholesterol and LDL (low-density, "bad" cholesterol).	Excessive omega-6 fats, if they are derived from processed or hydrogenated oils, are biochemically impotent.	corn, soybean, sunflower, and safflower oil

FAT AT A GLANCE (continued)

Type of Fat	U.S. Department of Agriculture Recommendations		Why Eat More	Why Eat Less	Sources
	1,500 Cal./Day Diet	2,000 Cal./Day Diet			
Omega-3 fats Current average: too low a proportion of omega-3 fats.	Ideally, you should eat omega-3s and omega-6s at a ratio of 2:1, omega-3s over omega-6s, then after 3 to 9 months, 1:1.		Contains linolenic acid, another essential fatty acid, which may prevent abnormal heart rhythms, boost the immune system, lower dangerous blood clotting, and play a role in brain and eye development.	To correct the balance between omega-3 and omega-6.	fish oil, flaxseed, walnuts, cold-water fish such as salmon, herring, and mackerel
Polyunsaturated Current overall average is low: only about 7% of daily calories. Any increase should be in omega-3 fats only.	17 gr. up to 10%	22 gr. up to 10%	Any increase should be in polyunsaturated omega-3s only.	To keep omega-6 and omega-3 in balance.	raw nuts, seeds, legumes, corn, and leafy greens

FAT AT A GLANCE (continued)

Type of Fat	U.S. Department of Agriculture Recommendations		Why Eat More	Why Eat Less	Sources
	1,500 Cal./Day Diet	2,000 Cal./Day Diet			
Saturated Current average is high: 12% of daily calories—over 50% more than recommended!	13 gr. 8% or less of total calories	18 gr. 8% or less of total calories		Increased risk of heart disease, colon and prostate cancer.	meat, poultry, whole-milk dairy products (butter, cream, whole milk, cheese), lard, coconut oil, palm and palm kernel oil
Trans Fatty Acids, Trans Fat Current average: Even at just over 2% of total calories, experts believe we should consume far, far less.	Eat as little as possible.		No reason to eat more.	Increased total cholesterol and LDLs ("bad" cholesterol). In very large amounts, trans fatty acids may also suppress good HDLs. High trans-fat intake may be linked to increased risk of breast cancer and gallstones.	shortening, stick margarine; packaged snacks, cookies, crackers, candy, and baked goods; pastries; deep-fried food, such as french fries; all products listing "hydrogenated" or "partially hydrogenated" oils in their ingredients (such as most commercial peanut butters)

THE GOOD NEWS ABOUT CARBOHYDRATES

Should you be avoiding carbohydrates and increasing your intake of fat and protein—the two types of food almost all of us should be eating less of? In my opinion, no. A calorie is a calorie, and gram for gram, carbohydrates contain the same number of calories as protein, and half as many as fat. Complex carbohydrates—from whole grains, fruits, vegetables, and beans—are an integral, irreplaceable component of a healthy diet. Here's why:

- **COMPLEX-CARBOHYDRATE FOODS SATISFY MORE THAN JUST HUNGER.** The sharp crunch of a fresh apple, the comforting texture of warm baked sweet potato, the smell of whole-grain toast: These are just a few of the pleasures of eating. Diets that call for drastic reductions in complex-carbohydrate foods are the most likely to provoke the cravings that make dieters feel deprived and on the verge of losing control.

- **YOUR MIND AND YOUR BODY NEED COMPLEX CARBOHYDRATES TO FUNCTION WELL.** Complex carbohydrates are the most easily and quickly metabolized form of food, and essential if you need to keep your energy and your blood-sugar level up throughout the day. See the box below for the carbs that rate lowest on the glycemic index, which means they offer a steady supply of blood sugar, boosting energy and blocking cravings.

- **FRUITS AND VEGETABLES ARE THE BEST NATURAL SOURCE OF VITAMINS, MINERALS, AND A HOST OF CHEMICALS THAT PROTECT AGAINST CANCER, HEART DISEASE, AND OTHER DISEASES.** Even though supplements may be indicated in certain situations (see "Do You Need Additional Vitamins and Minerals?," page 173), it's still best to obtain the bulk of your vitamins, minerals, antioxidants, and phytochemicals from real food. The reason is that some studies show that vitamins and other chemicals do not always confer the same protective benefit when isolated and taken in supplement form as they do when eaten in food. No one is sure why this is, although it seems likely that each food also contains other vitamins and chemicals that may enhance the effect of the others (see below).

- **COMPLEX-CARBOHYDRATE FOODS ARE THE BEST SOURCES OF DIETARY FIBER.** Dietary fiber is essential to day-to-day well-being and prevention of some forms of cancer and other diseases. High-fat, high-protein, low-carbohydrate diets are dangerously low in fiber, another reason why people on them often complain of feeling sluggish and not themselves.

Carbohydrates: The Best Sources of Anticancer Chemicals

Restrict carbohydrates and you miss a range of foods rich in chemicals that are now recognized as having anticancer properties.

PROTECTIVE CHEMICAL	CARBOHYDRATE SOURCES
allylic sulfides	garlic, onions
anthocyanins	bilberries, blueberries
catechins	berries
ellagic acid	blackberries, grapes, strawberries
flavonoids	berries, broccoli, cabbage, carrots, citrus fruits, cucumbers, eggplant, parsley, peppers, soy products, squash, tomatoes, yams
glucoraphanin	broccoli sprouts
indoles	broccoli, cabbage, cauliflower, mustard greens
isoflavones	beans, legumes, peanuts, peas
isothiocyanates	horseradish, mustard, radishes
lignans	flaxseed, walnuts
limonoids	citrus fruits
lycopene	red grapefruit, tomatoes

PROTECTIVE CHEMICAL	CARBOHYDRATE SOURCES *(continued)*
monoterpenes	basil, broccoli, carrots, citrus fruits, cucumbers, eggplant, mint, parsley, peppers, squash, tomatoes, yams
omega-3 polyunsaturated fatty acids	flaxseed, walnuts
phenolic acids	berries, broccoli, cabbage, carrots, citrus fruits, eggplant, parsley, peppers, tomatoes
plant sterols	broccoli, cabbage, cucumbers, eggplant, grains, peppers, soy products, squash, tomatoes, yams
polyacetylene	parsley
protease inhibitors	soybeans
quercetin	grapes
quinones	rosemary
terpenes	citrus fruits
triterpenoids	licorice root

What's Wrong with Pasta?

For most of us, nothing. But that's not the line being spouted by numerous popular diet gurus and best-selling diet books. The latest theory is that people gain weight because of what combinations of food they eat, not how much. This isn't the first time carbohydrates (in earlier decades referred to, unappetizingly, as "starch") have been banished from Fad Dietville. Only now carbohydrates are the villain in a syndrome known as insulin resistance.

Insulin resistance is real. It occurs in people whose bodies cannot regulate blood insulin levels. Instead of signaling the pancreas to stop producing insulin once the demand has been met, people who are insulin resistant have cells that don't seem to register "full," so the pancreas just keeps pumping out more insulin. Eventually the pancreas simply can't produce enough insulin, which means the glycogen in the blood has no way to get to your hungry cells, setting off a chain of events that can result in heart disease, kidney disease, and other serious health problems. While no one knows exactly what causes diabetes, it seems there is a genetic predisposition, and that eating a high-fat diet, being overweight, and not exercising regularly increases the likelihood that the disease will manifest itself. Experts estimate that half of the people who have non-insulin-dependent (also known as Type II or adult-onset) diabetes do not realize they have it, though it is easily diagnosed through blood tests.

As science learns more about the possible role of insulin in diabetes and heart disease, it seems there may be cause for concern for some people. Exactly who may be at risk is still a subject of debate. Until your doctor has determined that you are indeed insulin resistant, you should get the bulk of your daily calories from healthy, complex-carbohydrate foods.

The Best of the Good Carbohydrates

Not all complex carbohydrates are created equal. We used to divide carbohydrates between simple (usually thought of as sweet, sometimes refined, such as chocolate or fruit) and complex (usually thought to be high in fiber, high in starch, and low in sweetness). It would seem to make sense that a food with a higher percentage of sugar would boost blood sugar more dramatically than, for instance, plain rice. But beginning in the late 1970s, scientists put carbohydrates to the test and discovered some surprising facts. Out of this research, they developed the glycemic index, which essentially measures the degree to which a food prompts a quick, dramatic rise in blood sugar. The lower the food's index, the better it is for maintaining the steady, constant blood-sugar level that keeps you energized and blocks cravings. The higher the food's GI, the more likely it is to set off that rush-crash cycle that leaves you feeling tired, irritable, and hungrier than before.

Contrary to popular belief, you cannot determine a food's glycemic index standing based on taste alone, because ice cream and a hamburger roll rate the same 60 on the scale. Other surprising pairs sharing the same glycemic index: plain macaroni and sponge cake, brown rice and oatmeal cookies, popcorn and fruit cocktail, carrots and Life Savers candy. This doesn't mean that carrots are no better for you than candy, or that you should avoid foods with a high GI. Doing so would mean eliminating many important sources of vitamins, minerals, fiber, and other nutrients. The glycemic index is strictly a ranking of foods according to their ability to cause an insulin response in your bloodstream. It's an instant guide telling you what foods you can have in small, large, or average quantities.

LOW GI	MODERATE GI	HIGH GI
skim or whole milk, yogurt—low-fat plain or artificially sweetened and with fruit	cheese pizza, macaroni and cheese	
apples, apricots, cherries, grapefruit, kiwis, oranges, pears, plums	bananas, fruit cocktail, grapefruit juice, grapes, mangoes, orange juice, pineapple, pineapple juice, raisins	watermelon
black-eyed peas, butter beans, chickpeas, dried peas, lentils, lima beans, peanuts	black bean soup, green peas, popcorn	
hominy	beets, boiled white potatoes, sweet potatoes	baked potatoes, carrots, french fries, mashed potatoes, parsnips, pumpkin
custard pudding, peanut M&Ms, milk chocolate	angel food cake, ice cream, oatmeal cookies, pound cake	donuts, jelly beans, tofu frozen dessert
sausage		
instant rice, fettuccine, spaghetti	couscous, croissants, gnocchi, rye bread, wild rice	bagels, Cheerios, cornflakes, Cream of Wheat, pretzels, rice cakes

THE SUPER FOODS

Remember this: It's easier to eat right when you eat the right things. Every bite you take is an opportunity to treat your body really well. Does this mean you should never enjoy food again? No. Realistically, it would be impossible, not to mention boring, to refuse every food that "fails" the supernutrition test. Instead, add more of these "multi-tasking" foods to your diet as a form of "nutrition insurance." Calorie for calorie, super foods make healthy eating a snap.

WHAT TO EAT	WHAT'S IN IT FOR YOU	WHY EAT MORE
almonds, unsalted, unroasted, raw	*high in vitamin E, magnesium, potassium, calcium, folacin, B$_2$, and include zinc, copper, iron, phosphorus, and selenium*	*Almonds are 20 percent protein and less than 60 percent fat, all poly-unsaturated. They also contain amygdalin (laetrile), which may have an anticarcinogenic effect on cells, and linoleic acid, an essential fatty acid our bodies cannot produce.*
beans	*high in fiber, protein, and iron (half a cup supplies 10 percent of your RDA of iron), and include some B vitamins*	*At about 100 calories per 1/2 cup, 7 grams of protein, and 7 grams of fiber, beans are a nutritional bonanza. A serving of beans combined with rice is a complete protein. Soak beans overnight and discard that water before cooking in fresh water; this eliminates their gas-producing properties.*
broccoli sprouts	*high in vitamin A, vitamin C, folacin, potassium, phosphorus, magnesium, iron, and calcium, plus a concentrated amount of the phytochemical glucoraphanin*	*Broccoli sprouts, the early broccoli plant, are cruciferous vegetables, long thought to have anticancer properties. Glucoraphanin, which sprouts have 20 to 50 times more of than mature broccoli, neutralizes carcinogens before they inflict the damage on DNA that results in cancer.*
cereal, high-bran, low-sugar, and low-fat	*fiber, vitamins, and minerals (depending on brand and type)*	*Eating cereal is one of the easiest ways to get your RDA of many important vitamins and minerals, and meet your daily fiber requirements. Fiber has been shown to reduce the risk of colorectal, breast, and uterine cancers.*

WHAT TO EAT	WHAT'S IN IT FOR YOU	WHY EAT MORE (continued)
eggs, prepared with little or no fat	high in vitamin K, selenium, and riboflavin, plus 6 to 7 grams of protein each	At just 70 calories, a hard-boiled egg is truly a food of wonder—despite its reputation for raising cholesterol levels (see "The Good Egg," page 138). Eggs are inexpensive, versatile, and easily added to other foods. If you're concerned about antibiotics, hormones, and pesticides, buy organic.
flaxseed oil	omega-3 fatty acids such as alpha-linolenic acid and omega-6 acids such as linoleic acid; linolenic is the most important essential fatty acid	It promotes a healthy cardiovascular system, skin, prostate, and keeps joints well lubricated. Flaxseed oil can also help your body break down and eliminate body fat (see "Flax Facts," page 233).
garlic, fresh, not as a supplement	allylic sulfides (also in onions), which help to neutralize carcinogenic substances by activating enzymes that "disable" them	In addition to garlic's anticarcinogenic properties, it is a potent antioxidant, with the ability to prevent blood clots, fight bacteria, boost the immune system, and lower blood pressure.
oats, cooked	complex carbohydrates, soluble fiber; instant or flavored varieties are iron and vitamin fortified	Low in fat, high in carbohydrates, oats provide a satisfying meal that sticks with you for hours. Soluble fiber has been proven to lower blood cholesterol. Made with skim milk, oatmeal is a complete protein.
salmon	high in protein and omega-3 fatty acids; canned salmon, eaten with the bones, can provide 20 percent of your daily calcium requirement	Salmon's omega-3 acids can reduce your risk of heart attack, stroke, and arteriosclerosis. Fatty fish such as salmon may also help prevent breast cancer.

WHAT TO EAT	WHAT'S IN IT FOR YOU	WHY EAT MORE (continued)
soybeans (includes products such as oil, tempeh, tofu, soybean sprouts)	*a lot of protein with little fat, little sodium, and few calories; makes a complete protein when served with a complementary incomplete protein source, such as rice*	Soy contains genistein, a compound that's been proven to block the new blood vessels cancerous tumors form to get their blood supply. Genistein also blocks the estrogen receptors on estrogen-sensitive tissue, such as breast tissue. Soybeans also contain numerous other substances that prevent or inhibit the formation of cancer cells.
tomato sauce (and paste)	*vitamin C, vitamin A, and lycopene, a powerful antioxidant, all in a food that's low in calories, inexpensive, and very versatile; sauces and pastes are more nutritionally dense than fresh tomatoes, because they're concentrated*	The anticancer properties of lycopene are indisputable. Studies show a correlation between tomato sauce consumption and reductions in rates of cervical and prostate cancer. Lycopene may also be effective in preventing heart disease.
yogurt, active culture (not frozen)	*between 25% and 45% of your daily requirements for calcium, riboflavin, protein; active cultures of beneficial bacteria*	Nonfat and low-fat yogurts deliver a lot of protein and calcium for the calories. Studies have shown yogurt to be effective in boosting the immune system against bacteria, viruses, and possibly even cancer (so far just in mice). People who eat yogurt regularly have been found to suffer fewer colds, sinus infections, and hayfever. Yogurt with live L. acidophilus cultures has been shown to be effective against vaginitis, or yeast infections.

THE SUPER PRODUCE

We all know we should eat our fruits and veggies, because they're good for us. But some are just a little bit better than others at delivering a wide range of nutrients. Here are the produce superstars.

ESSENTIAL NUTRIENTS AND WHAT THEY DO	APRICOT	BROCCOLI	CABBAGE	CANTALOUPE	CARROT	CRANBERRY	KALE	KIWI	LEMON	MANGO	ORANGE	PAPAYA	SPINACH	TOMATO
vitamin A: for vision; general cell health; boosting immunity; healthy skin, hair, bones, teeth, and mucous membranes; reproduction		•		•	•		•						•	•
vitamin B_6: for creation of hemo-globin (red blood cells); regulation of myriad biochemical processes, including blood glucose levels		•		•									•	
beta-carotene: for protecting cells as an antioxidant	•			•						•	•	•	•	

ESSENTIAL NUTRIENTS AND WHAT THEY DO (continued)	APRICOT	BROCCOLI	CABBAGE	CANTALOUPE	CARROT	CRANBERRY	KALE	KIWI	LEMON	MANGO	ORANGE	PAPAYA	SPINACH	TOMATO
vitamin C: for healthy capillaries, bones, and teeth; formation of collagen; for boosting immunity		•	•	•		•	•	•	•	•	•	•	•	•
calcium: for strong, healthy bones, teeth, cell membranes; blood clotting; muscle contraction; activation of enzymes for biochemical processes		•					•		•				•	
folic acid: for red blood cell formation; synthesizing genetic material		•	•	•							•		•	
iron: for red blood cell formation; as a component of enzymes and proteins; for supplying oxygen to cells													•	
vitamin K: for blood clotting; bone health		•											•	

ESSENTIAL NUTRIENTS AND WHAT THEY DO (continued)	APRICOT	BROCCOLI	CABBAGE	CANTALOUPE	CARROT	CRANBERRY	KALE	KIWI	LEMON	MANGO	ORANGE	PAPAYA	SPINACH	TOMATO
lycopene: an anti-oxidant														•
magnesium: for maintaining electrolyte balance; proper metabolism of calcium and glucose; healthy nerves; manufacture of proteins	•	•								•			•	
pantothenic acid: for metabolism of carbohydrates, proteins, fats; formation of hormones		•								•	•			
potassium: for healthy fluid and electrolyte balance; metabolism of carbohydrates, proteins, fats; nerve impulse transmission; muscle contraction	•			•						•	•	•	•	•

ESSENTIAL NUTRIENTS AND WHAT THEY DO (continued)	APRICOT	BROCCOLI	CABBAGE	CANTALOUPE	CARROT	CRANBERRY	KALE	KIWI	LEMON	MANGO	ORANGE	PAPAYA	SPINACH	TOMATO
riboflavin (B$_2$): for healthy mucous membranes; metabolism of food		•											•	
zinc: for boosting immunity; creation of enzymes necessary to bio-chemical processes											•			

THERE'S NO SUCH THING AS A "BAD" FRUIT OR VEGETABLE

For decades dieters have been avoiding potatoes and bananas because they were "too starchy," dried fruits because of their concentrated sugar content, and avocados because they're high in fat. This is a big mistake, because each of these foods deserves a place in your kitchen. Potatoes and bananas are rich in potassium, dried fruits provide fiber, and avocados, though calorie-dense, are an excellent source of monounsaturated fat (only hazelnuts have a higher concentration of this cholesterol-fighting fat) and have powerful antioxidant properties. Remember: How "good" or "bad" any food is depends on how we eat it.

NUTS ABOUT NUTS

Here's a tip that breaks every diet book taboo: Eat more nuts. Yes, I know they are dense in calories and in fat, but that doesn't mean they shouldn't be part of your diet. Several large, long-term studies have established that people who eat nuts in moderation (that is, they consume nuts while keeping their total fat intake at healthy levels) reduced their risk of heart attack by up to 50 percent. That's because nuts are rich in the best kind of fat, monounsaturated. They contain the antioxidant vitamin E, and some also boast omega-3 fatty acids—both heart protectors—in addition to protein, fiber, zinc, magnesium, and copper. Studies have also shown that people who eat nuts several times a week have lower cholesterol levels.

Still a little hesitant to grant the long-maligned nut a place on your plate? The key is to treat nuts as real food sources, not just snacks. You can add nuts to your diet without adding pounds to yourself by forgoing the oily snack varieties and the rich snack concoctions (such as trail mixes and ambrosia) you know you'll be tempted to eat too much of. Instead, sprinkle nuts on vegetables, add them to baked goods, stir fries, and salads. Regard them as a protein source, like meat or legumes, and use them sparingly. Also remember that not all nuts are created equal, calorie-wise. An ounce of chestnuts contains less than a single gram of fat and 70 calories. An ounce of cashews delivers over twice the calories and a whopping 13 grams of fat. The healthiest nuts are walnuts, almonds, chestnuts, and macadamia nuts.

THE WONDER BERRIES AND OTHER SMALL FRUIT

They're the munchkins of the fruit world, juicy little jewels in red, blue, and purple. Too often relegated to garnish duty or buried in sugary pies, jellies, and jams, berries, cherries, and grapes aren't usually included among the superstar fruits like oranges, papayas, kiwis, and bananas. But there's a lot to like about these tiny fruits, and good reason to make room for them.

- **ANTHOCYANINS.** These are the antioxidants that give blueberries and cherries their dark color. Of all fruits, blueberries have the highest concentration of cancer-fighting anthocyanins. In the test tube, blueberry anthocyanins (and those from bilberries) crippled an enzyme that causes the rapid cell division typical of malignant tumors.

- **ANTIBACTERIAL AND ANTIVIRAL ACTIVITY.** We've long known that cranberry juice can prevent and help vanquish bacterial bladder infections by making the cells the bacteria hang on to less hospitable. We now know that blueberries, which grow on bushes of the same genus, have a similar effect on bladder infections. Blueberries are also effective against *E. coli* bacteria. In Sweden, doctors have traditionally prescribed dried blueberries (1/3 ounce) to treat diarrhea in children. (Fresh blueberries are not as effective as dried.) Raspberries, strawberries, and red grapes also have antiviral and antibacterial properties.

- **A NATURAL SOURCE OF CLOT-BLOCKING SALICYLATES AND RESVERATROL.** Cranberries, blueberries, raspberries, cherries, and strawberries are all rich in salicylates, the active ingredient in aspirin that helps prevent the clotting that can lead to heart attacks and strokes. A 1998 study from the University of Wisconsin Medical School found that purple grape juice may be stronger than aspirin in reducing blood clots in healthy people. Found in red grape skin, another chemical called resveratrol produces a similar action and promotes high-density lipid (HDL, or "good") cholesterol.

- **CANCER-PREVENTING CHEMICALS.** Foods that "fight" cancer have not yet been found. But berries are rich in several chemicals that are known to interrupt cellular processes conducive to cancer: catechins (antioxidants), flavonoids (which inhibit cancer-promoting hormones), and phenolic acids (which work as antioxidants, inhibit the formation of carcinogenic nitrosamines, and disrupt enzyme activity crucial to cancer-cell growth). Grapes contain another anticancer chemical, quercetin, an antioxidant.

- **VITAMIN C.** Blackberries, cherries, and strawberries are all rich in vitamin C, which blocks the formation of carcinogenic nitrosamines in the digestive tract.

DON'T SUBSTITUTE JUICE FOR FRUIT

Compared to many other beverages—such as iced tea, soft drinks, sports drinks, coffee, and juice drinks—100 percent fruit juice is without a doubt the healthier choice. But if you're trying to cut your calories and increase your daily fiber intake, skip the juice and go for its source fruit. At over 100 calories per 8-ounce serving, fruit juices are not very filling.

SHOPPING SMARTER

We take it on faith that fruits and vegetables are good for us, and they are. But not all produce is created equal. Make these wise choices the next time you shop:

CHOOSE ...	OVER ...	BECAUSE ...
almonds	peanuts, cashews, and hazelnuts	almonds have: • lower fat content than most other nuts; • higher protein content—about 20 percent—than other nuts; • low sodium; • high levels of vitamin E, calcium, zinc, and magnesium.
broccoli sold in "modified atmosphere packaging" (a plastic that slows food deterioration)	unpackaged fresh broccoli	modified atmosphere packaging preserves almost all the vitamin C, while broccoli packaged other ways loses up to 76 percent.
broccoli sprouts	broccoli	the sprouts have 20 to 50 times the cancer-fighting phytochemical glucoraphanin of mature broccoli.
cantaloupe	honeydew, watermelon	cantaloupe contains more beta-carotene.
green onions (scallions)	yellow onions	green onions are higher in vitamins A and C and iron.
guavas	mangoes	guavas have 6 times the vitamin C.
mangoes	guavas	mangoes have more than 4 times the vitamin A.

CHOOSE . . .	OVER . . .	BECAUSE . . . *(continued)*
orange juice	apple juice	an 8-ounce glass of orange juice gives you: • twice your RDA for vitamin C; • potassium and folic acid.
orange sweet potatoes	yellow sweet potatoes	orange sweet potatoes have more beta-carotene.
pink or red grapefruit	white grapefruit	though all are excellent sources of vitamin C, pink and red grapefruit also contain the antioxidant beta-carotene.
red peppers	green peppers	a 3½-ounce serving gives you: • twice the vitamin C; • more beta-carotene than green peppers • over 100 percent of the RDA for vitamin A.
romaine lettuce	iceberg lettuce	romaine lettuce has: • 6 times the vitamin C; • 5 to 10 times the beta-carotene.
snow peas	shelled green peas	a 3½-ounce serving gives you: • 100 percent of your RDA for vitamin C; • almost double the calcium of green peas (which are higher in B vitamins and protein).
strawberries	raspberries	strawberries are higher in vitamins A and C, iron, and potassium.

FOOD ADDITIVES: WHEN TO SAY NO

How much should you worry about the 5 pounds of nonnutrient food additives each one of us consumes every year? Among the health-conscious, the terms *food additives* and *preservatives* have become another way of saying *poison*. Yet unless you can avail yourself of a totally organic diet of fresh foods and live without packaged or precooked foods, it's virtually impossible not to encounter at least a few. Each year, we consume over a hundred pounds of sugar, corn syrup, and salt. Many other additives are nutrients, such as vitamins, that are added to replace those lost during shipping, processing, or storage, or to enhance a food that otherwise does not contain them (for example, the vitamin C added to apple juice).

If you believe that the FDA can protect us completely from suspect or potentially dangerous additives, you're wrong. If, on the other hand, you believe that every ingredient that you can't pronounce or define presents an imminent danger, you're wrong too. *Natural* does not automatically mean safe; *synthetic* does not always mean dangerous. For example, before widespread refrigeration and the advent of chemical meat preservatives, most meat was preserved with salt. Though salt is undeniably a "natural" substance, during the 1930s, it contributed to an epidemic that made stomach cancer the leading cause of cancer death for men, and the third for women. (Today, despite our consuming many times more "unnatural," chemical preservatives, stomach cancer has dropped to become the sixteenth most common fatal cancer, and a substantial proportion of those cases are linked to smoking and alcohol.)

For many of us, "can't live with 'em, can't live without 'em" captures our additive predicament. Additives (namely antioxidants and chelating agents) not only help preserve food so that it has a longer shelf life, but also keep food looking, smelling, and tasting better (as emulsifiers, flavor enhancers, or thickening agents). Yes, as critics claim, longer shelf life helps fatten food-store and food-manufacturers' profits. But it also protects consumers from getting packaged foods that are rancid or dangerous to consume, and in some cases makes it possible for consumers to eat a diet that includes foods not locally grown or produced.

So where is the middle ground? Some additives are dangerous and should be avoided. In most cases that's easy to do, since many of the most worrisome additives, such as artificial sweeteners and artificial colors, are used in the foods we should be eating less of anyway (junk diet dessert foods, diet sodas, baked goods, candy, cookies, ice cream, processed meat products). Based on information compiled by the Center for Science in the Public Interest, here is a list of those you can relax about.

Coloring Agents:
annatto
beta-carotene (your body converts this to vitamin A)
betaine
ferrous gluconate

Emulsifiers, Conditioners, Thickeners:
alginates, propylene glycol alginate
calcium propionate, sodium propionate
calcium stearoyl lactate, sodium stearoyl lactylate
carrageenan
casein, sodium caseinate
citric acid, sodium citrate
EDTA
gelatin
glycerin, glycerol
gums
lactic acid
lecithin
monoglycerides, diglycerides
phosphoric acid, phosphates (also used as nutrients and color stabilizers)
polysorbate 60
sodium carboxymethyl cellulose (CMC)
sorbitan monostearate
starch
starch, modified

Flavor Enhancers:
fumaric acid
malic acid
methionine (an essential amino acid)
vanillin, ethyl vanillin

Nutrients:
alpha-tocopherol (vitamin E)

beta-carotene
thiamin mononitrate (vitamin B$_1$)

Preservatives, Including Antioxidants:
ascorbic acid (vitamin C), sodium ascorbate
calcium propionate
erythorbic acid
propionic acid
sodium benzoate
sodium carboxymethyl cellulose (CMC)
sorbic acid, potassium sorbate

The Additives You Should Always Avoid

1. **ACESULFAME K** (also known as acesulfame potassium): artificial sweetener that's 200 times sweeter than sugar. It's found in diet soda drinks, baked goods, gelatin desserts, and chewing gum.

2. **ARTIFICIAL COLORS:** Only a few must be listed individually, so you never know if you're getting one of the food dyes whose safety is questionable. Be on the lookout for these: Blue 1, Blue 2, Green 3, Red 3, Red 40, Yellow 5, Yellow 6.

3. **ASPARTAME:** an artificial sweetener better known under the trade names NutraSweet and Equal; found in a wide range of sugar-free diet foods.

4. **BHA** (butylated hydroxyanisole): preservative, antioxidant, often found in the same products as BHT (see below): vegetable oil, cereal, chewing gum, potato chips, and other snack foods.

5. **BHT** (butylated hydroxytoluene): preservative, antioxidant; see above.

6. **OLESTRA** (Olean): a fat substitute found in lower-fat chips and crackers.

7. **POTASSIUM BROMATE:** increases the volume of baked goods; found in breads and rolls. It has been banned virtually everywhere in the world but Japan and the United States.

8. **PROPYL GALLATE:** antioxidant, preservative. This is used in meat products, vegetable oil, chicken-soup base, and chewing gum.

9. **SACCHARIN:** an artificial sweetener best known under the trade name Sweet'n Low is 350 times sweeter than sugar. It's found in sugar-free diet products and soft drinks.

10. **SODIUM NITRATE:** a preservative also used to enhance flavoring and coloring; appears most often in processed meat products (bacon, cold cuts and luncheon meats, hot dogs, etc.) and smoked fish.

11. **SODIUM NITRITE:** a preservative also used to enhance flavoring and coloring; see above.

Additives You May Be Sensitive To

This is by no means a complete list, since it's possible to be sensitive to any food or additive. These are the additives to which a notable number of people have reported sensitivity:

- **ARTIFICIAL COLORINGS,** especially Yellow 5. Artificial colorings are everywhere, it seems, but most likely to be found in food you can live without: candy, baked goods, cake mixes and prepared frostings, soft drinks, gelatin, pudding, soft drinks, juice drinks, processed foods, processed meat products.

- **ASPARTAME** (See above).

- **CAFFEINE** is a stimulant that occurs naturally in coffee, tea, and chocolate. It is also added to soft drinks, bottled water, and over-the-counter preparations for headache and premenstrual discomfort. Watch for it also in products flavored with coffee or chocolate.

- **CARMINE, OR COCHINEAL,** is a red dye made from beetles. It's found in all manner of junk food that needs to be colored purple, red, or pink.

- **GUM TRAGACANTH,** a thickening agent found in ice cream, baked goods, salad dressings, and some reduced-fat products.

- **HVP, HYDROLYZED VEGETABLE PROTEIN,** is a flavor enhancer that contains MSG. It's found in prepared soups, sauce mixes, hot dogs, canned beef stew, and other canned meat products.

- **LACTOSE,** sugar found in milk; only a problem if you suffer lactose intolerance. Lactose is used in whipped topping mix, packaged breakfast pastries, and other packaged goods.

- **MONOSODIUM GLUTAMATE (MSG)** may also be an ingredient in other additives, such as hydrolyzed vegetable protein and modified food starch.

- **QUININE,** a flavoring found in quinine water, tonic water, and bitter lemon. It may cause birth defects.

- **SULFITES (SODIUM BISULFITE, SULFUR DIOXIDE)** are found in dried fruit, wines, fresh and frozen shrimp, dried, fried, or frozen potatoes. Allergic reactions to sulfites range from mild to severe, especially in asthmatics. Twelve people are known to have suffered fatal reactions to sulfites.

Getting Even More: Vitamins, Minerals, and Supplements

5.

Jason, in his mid-twenties, was fortunate to grow up in a family where health and fitness were woven into daily life. Unlike most of his friends in law school, Jason ate well, exercised regularly—if not as often as he wished—and generally took very good care of himself. When he got his first job, however, the time to exercise and to prepare good meals for himself was limited. He rarely left his office until after seven at night, and he often worked at home until nearly midnight. Amazingly, Jason was still eating better than most people and getting out for a good run at least three times a week. But he felt tired, run-down, and for the first time in his life was fighting a chronic sinus infection he just couldn't seem to shake. Clearly, he needed something else.

VITAMINS AND MINERALS: THE BASICS

Vitamins are organic (meaning they contain carbon) compounds and minerals are inorganic (meaning they don't contain carbon) elements that are present in food and are necessary for health and life itself. Without vitamins and minerals, our bodies cannot "process" the raw materials of proteins, carbohydrates, and fats to create everything that sustains life: energy, hormones, blood cells, new tissue, DNA, neurochemicals, enzymes, and immune cells. Perhaps equally important, some vitamins and minerals cannot be metabolized properly or used efficiently in the absence of others; the relationship between vitamin D and calcium is a good example of this synergy. This is why people rarely have a single, easily diagnosed deficiency, and why it may not be particularly useful to memorize the specific contribution each vitamin or mineral makes to your health. Instead, be sure that you get the Recommended Daily Allowance (RDA) with adjustments for the demands and stresses of your life. (Beware, however, of megadoses; see "Megadoses: Getting More—or Less—Than You Bargained For," page 193.) See also specific sections in this chapter on vitamins C and E, calcium, and iron.

WHAT YOU NEED TO KNOW ABOUT VITAMINS AND MINERALS

- **RDA.** The Recommended Daily Allowance levels, which you may be most familiar with, were established more than twenty-five years ago and most recently revised in 1989. Originally, these reflected the amounts of essential nutrients then deemed adequate to prevent disease or the adverse effects of deficiency in healthy people. As knowledge broadens about the roles nutrients play in maintaining health and preventing disease, many of these values are being revised.

- **DAILY VALUES** The Daily Values, the numbers referred to on Nutrition Facts labels, are based on the Reference Daily Intakes (RDI), a newer set of reference values. The Institute of Medicine's Food and Nutrition Board, in partnership with Health Canada, is currently studying the role of a wider range of nutrients and is expected to issue a full set of revised RDIs sometime in the year 2000. In the meantime, it will be issuing new findings as they emerge.

- **VITAMINS ARE DIVIDED INTO TWO CLASSES ACCORDING TO HOW THEY ARE METABOLIZED: FAT-SOLUBLE AND WATER-SOLUBLE.**

  Fat-soluble vitamins—A, D, E, and K—cannot be absorbed in the digestive tract without the presence of dietary fat. These vitamins are also stored in body fat, so if you don't meet your requirements today, but did in the past several days, you're fine. The downside of storing vitamins is that they can build up to toxic levels. This is why you should never megadose on fat-soluble vitamins.

  Water-soluble vitamins—B complex and C—need to be replenished daily. B_6 (pyridoxine) is the exception, because it can remain in the body and build up to toxic levels. Contrary to popular belief, however, it is possible to "overdose" on them. Water-soluble vitamins tend to be less stable in food and are easily "lost" by improper storage or cooking.

- **MINERALS.** Minerals are classified as either macrominerals (calcium, chloride, magnesium, phosphorus, potassium, sodium, and sulfur) or microminerals, also known as trace minerals (chromium, copper, fluorine, iodine, iron, manganese, molybdenum, and zinc). A balanced diet provides most of the minerals you need, with the possible exception of zinc and, in certain cases, iron. RDAs for some minerals are not set because there is a question of how much is necessary or, in the case of a few, whether they are necessary at all.

RECOMMENDED DIETARY ALLOWANCES (RDAs) FOR ADULT WOMEN, AGE 19 TO 50

The RDAs are the levels of intake of essential nutrients sufficient to maintain good nutrition in practically all healthy people in the United States. The % Daily Value (DV) information on the "Nutrition Facts" label tells consumers about the individual food's contribution toward a 2,000-calorie-a-day diet. The Daily Values for vitamins and minerals are based on the U.S. RDAs issued by the National Academy of Sciences. The Food and Drug Administration (FDA), which is responsible for label regulation, has not established a DV for all nutrients, and a listing on a product's Nutrition Facts for such nutrients is not mandatory. That's why it's good to have a basic knowledge of which foods are richest in specific important nutrients, such as calcium, iron, folate, and zinc. Your daily requirements for certain nutrients (for example, iron and thiamine) may be higher than the RDAs listed below. This chart is based on the 1989 RDAs for women age 19 to 50. Where the RDA for men differs, it is noted. You can find additional, age-specific nutrient information at the U.S. Department of Agriculture's website: http://www.nal.usda.gov.

The National Academy of Sciences' Institute of Medicine is in the process of reviewing current research and suggesting new guidelines. Among the previously released recommendations were calls for higher levels for calcium and folic acid, for example. A full set of revised guidelines is expected within the next few years. Unlike the RDAs, which are intended to maintain the proper nutrition of most people, these new allowances—currently known as the Dietary Reference Intakes (DRIs)—will shift the focus from deficiency prevention to promotion of health.

nutrient	RDA, women	notes
Fat-Soluble Vitamins		
vitamin A, I.U.	**4,000**	
vitamin D, I.U.	**400**	**600 for people over age 71 (1998)**
vitamin E, I.U.	**30**	
vitamin K, mcg.	**65**	
Water-Soluble Vitamins		
B_1, thiamine, mg.	**1.1**	
B_2, riboflavin, mg.	**1.3**	
B_3, niacin, mg. (NE)	**15**	
B_6, pyridoxinen, mg.	**1.6**	
B_9, folate, ug.	**180**	**400 mcg. (1998)**
B_{12}, cobalamin, ug.	**2.0**	
vitamin C, ascorbic acid, mg.	**60**	

nutrient	RDA, women	most recent National Academy of Sciences recommendations (date released)
Minerals and Trace Elements		
calcium, mg.	**800**	**increased to 1,000; 1,300 milligrams for women over**

nutrient	RDA, women	notes
		age 50 and others at risk for osteoporosis (1998)
copper, mg.	**1.5–3.0**	
iodine, mcg.	**150**	
iron, mg.	**15**	**for men, 10 mg. RDA**
magnesium, mg.	**280**	
phosphorus, mg.	**1,200**	**RDA 800, ages 25 to 50**
potassium, mg.	**no RDA**	**3,500 milligrams DV**
selenium, mcg.	**55**	**for men, 70 mcg. RDA**
zinc, mg.	**12**	

DO YOU NEED ADDITIONAL VITAMINS AND MINERALS?

Lifestyle, health, and activity can all make extraordinary nutritional demands. To meet them, consider these supplements:

IF YOU . . .	YOU MIGHT ADD . . .
drink alcohol (more than 2 drinks a day)	vitamin B complex vitamin C vitamin E
take antacids	calcium
take aspirin	vitamin C vitamin B complex
are breast-feeding	vitamin A vitamin E thiamine

IF YOU . . .	YOU MIGHT ADD . . . (continued)
are breast-feeding	riboflavin vitamin B complex vitamin D vitamin C niacin
smoke cigarettes	vitamin C vitamin E
drink coffee (more than 2 cups a day)	vitamin B complex beta-carotene
take oral contraceptives	vitamin B complex
diet or eat very low fat foods	a multiple vitamin with minerals
take diuretics	potassium magnesium zinc
don't get enough "good" fats, from olive oil, nuts, avocados	vitamin B complex vitamin C vitamin E
don't get enough green leafy vegetables	a multiple vitamin with minerals
are deficient in iron	See your doctor.
take laxatives	calcium and a multiple vitamin
are physically active	vitamin B complex iron

IF YOU . . .	YOU MIGHT ADD . . .
experience excessive amounts of stress	*vitamin B complex*
live in a crowded urban area	*vitamin C* *vitamin E* *beta-carotene*
are a vegetarian	*vitamin B complex,* *especially B$_{12}$, and a* *multiple vitamin*
are a vegetarian who does not eat dairy products	*as above, plus calcium*
are a woman over 35	*a multiple vitamin plus* *calcium and* *vitamin D* *vitamin E*

PICKING THE RIGHT BASIC MULTIVITAMIN AND MINERAL SUPPLEMENT

Even if you eat pretty well, you may feel you're better off with a little bit of nutritional "insurance" in the form of a multivitamin and mineral supplement. There are currently thousands of products out there, so how to choose? "Natural" or not? Tablets or capsules? Everything in one dose or several supplements spread out through the day? Megadoses across the board or the RDA? Expensive brands from the health food store or the line the discount drugstore carries? Here's everything you need to know.

- **START WITH THE BASICS.** You want a multiple vitamin and mineral supplement that is complete, with 100 percent of the RDA or DV for vitamins A, C, D, K, and the B complex, including niacin and folic acid, plus trace minerals such as boron, chromium, copper, manganese, selenium, and zinc.

- **SKIP THE IRON IF YOU DON'T NEED IT.** Unless your doctor has diagnosed an iron deficit, you may not need extra iron. If you're over thirty, be sure you've been tested for hemochromatosis before you supplement iron.

- **CONSULT YOUR DOCTOR.** If you are pregnant, lactating, or have a specific health condition, do not take any supplement without consulting your doctor.

- **HOW MUCH IS ENOUGH?** Generally, your multivitamin and mineral supplement should give you at least 100 percent of the Daily Value and no more than 300 percent. Refer to the chart on page 172. (Your vitamin labels may read "RDA"; it's the same as the DV.)

- **STRIVE FOR BALANCE.** Go for a multi that offers roughly the same percentage of the DV for each nutrient.

- **AVOID SPECIAL FORMULATIONS, ESPECIALLY THOSE THAT MAKE EXTRAVAGANT CLAIMS ABOUT THEIR POWER TO PREVENT DISEASE.** When it comes to vitamins, minerals, and other nutritional supplements, there is no authority with the power of the FDA looking over manufacturers' shoulders. Watch for terms like *balanced, high potency, revolutionary, complete*—they mean nothing. Read the label. Be especially wary of any supplement formulation that promises to prevent disease. If you read the fine print you'll probably see the word *may* at least once or a disclaimer to the effect that no one really knows if this substance is effective.

- **LOOK FOR THE USP (UNITED STATES PHARMACOPOEIA) SEAL OF APPROVAL.** But bear in mind that all this guarantees is that a supplement will dissolve within a certain period of time and that it in fact contains the nutrients in the amounts listed on the label.

- **SPEND YOUR MONEY WISELY.** Unless you have some dietary restrictions that require special formulations, you should be able to purchase your basic multi and a few supplements for about $15 to $20 a month. If you're spending more than that on the basics, check your labels again.

- **TAKE YOUR SUPPLEMENTS THE RIGHT WAY.** Taking certain nutritional supplements under the wrong conditions can compromise, even negate, their effectiveness. Make the most out of your supplements by getting into a routine that takes the following into account:

Supplement	Take it	How
multivitamin and minerals	with a whole glass of water and food	once a day
vitamin C take with iron	with food	once a day (for doses less than 500 mg.); if you take more than 500 mg., spread it out in several equal doses of 500 mg. or less
vitamin E do not take with iron	with food that contains some fat	once a day
calcium, magnesium do not take with other supplements	with dairy products, if possible	once or twice a day (depending on how many milligrams you're taking)
zinc do not take with dairy, coffee, tea, or wine	with meals that include nondairy protein	once a day

IRON: TOO MUCH OF A GOOD THING?

Iron is an essential trace mineral our bodies use to deliver oxygen to blood and muscle cells. Without iron, our bodies would not be able to carry out many basic, crucial biochemical functions, and the symptoms of anemia would appear in the form of fatigue, listlessness, muscle weakness, delayed healing, compromised immune function, dizziness, shortness of breath, and rapid heartbeat. Most of us grew up believing we were all at risk for "iron-poor blood," particularly premenopausal women, who need 50 percent (15 milligrams a day) more iron than men (10 milligrams). Pregnant and lactating women need three times as much (30 milligrams a day). But, in fact, newer evidence suggests that far fewer people than previously thought suffer from anemia due to iron deficiency. Most iron deficiency results from causes other than diet (namely, heavy menstrual bleeding and chronic bleeding in the gastrointestinal tract). Generally, women are more likely to suffer from iron deficiency; men more likely to suffer from iron overload.

Too Much Iron: The Dangers

When your body takes in more iron than it needs, the level of free radicals increases. Free radicals are oxygen molecules that contain unpaired electrons. These electrons essentially go out searching for a "mate" and damage healthy cells in the process. Too much free-radical damage is believed to heighten the risk for cancer. Antioxidants protect cells by blocking free radicals.

We already know that people who have a rare genetic disorder called hemochromatosis are at greater-than-average risk for heart disease, liver cancer, arthritis, diabetes, sterility, and impotence, among other conditions. People with hemochromatosis are generally advised to lower their iron intake, to not cook in iron pots and pans, and to avoid iron-enriched foods.

Hemochromatosis affects only about 1 in 200 to 250 people, but experts now believe that all adults over the age of thirty should be tested for it. It's not clear whether the risk of too much iron is as compelling for people without hemochromatosis, but given iron's known effects on free radicals, better to err on the side of caution. Besides, there's no demonstrated benefit in ingesting iron in quantities above the RDA.

Too Little Iron

If you are suffering any of the symptoms associated with anemia, ask your doctor to determine your iron level through a simple blood test. Then follow your doctor's recommendations for increasing the iron in your diet. Unless you have another health condition that is affecting your ability to ingest enough iron, are pregnant or nursing, or menstruate very heavily, you may not need a supplement. If an iron supplement is recommended, consider one made from vegetable sources, such as Floradix (available in health food stores); it's less likely to be constipating.

Getting the Right Amount

If you're not anemic or suffering from iron overload:

- **AVOID IRON SUPPLEMENTS.** Unless recommended by your doctor to address a specific iron deficiency (not just because he thinks a little extra iron is a good thing for everyone), find a multivitamin without iron. Most foods, except for oils, contain at least small quantities of iron. Fortified breakfast cereals range in iron content from 1 to 9 milligrams per serving. Read the label.

- **EXERCISE REGULARLY.** A program of regular exercise will help keep iron from building to excessive levels, as does donating blood.

- **EAT THE RIGHT AMOUNT OF IRON.** Meat, particularly livers and kidneys, are super sources of protein and iron. Three ounces of braised pork liver provide 15 milligrams of iron—100 percent of the RDA for women. However, most of us aren't avid organ eaters or are trying to cut down on meat, particularly beef (another rich source). See the chart below for other good sources of iron.

- **EAT IRON-RICH FOODS THE RIGHT WAY.** Generally, only a percentage of the iron you eat is actually absorbed by your body. Eating iron foods (or supplements) with foods containing vitamin C (or a supplement) in the same meal dramatically increases the amount of iron your body absorbs. Iron from meat (called "heme" iron) is more efficiently digested than that from nonmeat sources ("nonheme" iron). You absorb 15 to 30 percent of heme iron, and 5 percent of nonheme iron. Meals that combine both ensure better absorption of the nonheme iron. Eating iron-rich foods with whole eggs or tea can result in decreased absorption.

BEST SOURCES OF IRON

food	portion	iron, mg.
apricots, dried	10 halves	1.2
beef steak, tenderloin, broiled	3 oz.	2.6
cashews, dry roasted	1 oz.	1.7
chicken breast, roasted, with skin	half	1.0
clams, steamed	3 oz.	23.7
egg yolk, large	1	.06

food	portion	iron, mg. (continued)
figs, dried	5 large	1.2
kidney beans, dried, cooked	1/2 cup	2.0
kiwis, fresh	4 large	1.4
lentils, dried, cooked	1/2 cup	3.3
molasses, blackstrap	1 tbsp.	3.5
mussels, cooked	3 oz.	5.7
oatmeal, instant	1 packet	8.5
oysters, canned	3 oz.	5.7
peaches, dried	5 halves	2.6
pears, dried	5 halves	1.8
peas, green, cooked	1/2 cup	1.2
pine nuts, raw	1 oz.	2.6
pistachio nuts, dry roasted	2 oz.	1.8
potatoes, with skin, baked	1 large	1.4
prunes, dried	10	2.1
pumpkin seed kernels, roasted	1 oz.	4.2
raisins	1/2 cup	1.7

food	portion	iron, mg. (continued)
sardines, canned in tomato sauce	2	1.6
sauerkraut, canned, drained	1/2 cup	2.0
soybeans, dried, cooked	1/2 cup	4.4
soybeans, roasted	1/4 cup	1.5
spinach, cooked	1/2 cup	3.2
split peas, dried, cooked	1/2 cup	1.3
sunflower seed kernels, dried	1/4 cup	2.3
tofu, raw, firm	1/2 cup	13.0
tomato sauce, canned	1 cup	1.8
turkey, dark meat, roasted, with skin	3½ oz.	3.0
turkey, white meat, roasted, with skin	3½ oz.	1.4
turnip greens, cooked	1/2 cup	1.1
walnuts, dried	1 oz.	0.9
wheat cereal, Cream of Wheat, instant, cooked	1 cup	12.0

IRON AND THE BRAIN

Our brain cells are extremely sensitive to even the slightest drop in oxygen supply. Anytime you're deficient or low in iron, it affects oxygen delivery to the brain. Researchers in Indonesia found that women with low iron levels were less productive at work and at home.

VITAMIN C: THE FIRST "SUPERSTAR" NUTRIENT

Even people who are nutritionally illiterate know about vitamin C and its many powers, alleged and real. In 1970, it became the first "superstar" nutrient when Nobel Prize–winning chemist Dr. Linus Pauling claimed that vitamin C could prevent the common cold. Alas, controlled studies did not completely support Pauling's case (colds were milder, but not avoided). However, in the years since, vitamin C has emerged as more powerful than previously imagined. Known since the eighteenth century for its ability to prevent scurvy—a debilitating, crippling, potentially fatal nutritional deficiency common to sailors and poor people—vitamin C is now credited with the ability to lower blood pressure, control asthma and bronchitis, halt macular degeneration, and keep LDL (low-density, the "bad") cholesterol in check.

Because vitamin C is so plentiful in the average diet, there is some debate as to whether supplements are even necessary, since most of us easily get the RDA of 60 milligrams in a single orange or a little more than a half cup of broccoli. But is that enough? Given the overwhelmingly positive findings of most research into vitamin C's benefits and its low toxicity (it's water soluble, which means the body does not store it and it must be replenished daily), 200 milligrams is now considered a more reasonable daily amount. In 1999, researchers at the National Institutes of Health recommended that the daily allowance be increased but cautioned that anything more than 200 milligrams could increase the risk of kidney stones. You may consider becoming more conscientious about your vitamin C intake if you are concerned about any of the following:

- **BRUISING.** A telltale sign of vitamin C deficiency. Vitamin C is a key component of collagen, the protein that forms muscles, bones, cartilage, and skin. Collagen forms a protective sheath around blood vessels. (Chronic bruising should be brought to your doctor's attention, since it could indicate a more serious problem.)

- **CHRONIC INFECTIONS.** While vitamin C may not single-handedly wipe out the common cold, it is crucial to the immune system.

- **REDUCING YOUR RISK OF CANCER.** Over thirty studies have shown a link between diets high in vitamin C and reduced rates of cancer. Vitamin C is an antioxidant, and it also blocks the formation of carcinogenic nitrosamines.

- **KEEPING YOUR HEART HEALTHY.** Vitamin C reduces cholesterol through its antioxidant action. Its contribution to collagen production also keeps vessels pliable, healthy, and less prone to damage.

ARE ROSE HIPS A SUPERIOR SOURCE OF VITAMIN C?

Rose hips—the hard red berry-type fruit produced by some rose species—have long been hailed as a superior, natural source of vitamin C. Rose hips are used in teas, jellies, tablets, capsules, and liquid extracts. Milligram for milligram of ascorbic acid, rose hips may cost up to ten times more than other vitamin C products. Before you open your wallet, you should know that there's no evidence that vitamin C from rose hips is better for you than other forms. Some claim that because rose hips are "natural," the vitamin C is more easily absorbed, but that's really a nonissue, because C is plentiful and readily absorbed to begin with. As for the possible trace nutrients, such as phytochemicals, if they do exist, they have yet to be identified. Finally, read carefully. Just because a label says you're getting 100 milligrams of rose hips doesn't guarantee you're getting 100 milligrams of vitamin C.

BEST SOURCES OF VITAMIN C

food	portion	vitamin C, mg.
asparagus, cooked	1/2 cup	9.7
banana	medium	11
blackberries, fresh	1 cup	30
broccoli, cooked, chopped	1/2 cup	49
brussels sprouts, cooked	1/2 cup	35
cabbage, green, cooked, shredded	1/2 cup	15
cabbage, red, raw, shredded	1/2 cup	20
cantaloupe, diced	1 cup	65
cauliflower, cooked	1/2 cup	34
grapefruit	1/2 medium	44
grapefruit juice, from concentrate	1 cup	83
guava, raw	1	165
kale, cooked, chopped	1/2 cup	26
kiwi	1 medium	74
orange	1 medium	70
orange juice, fresh	1 cup	124
orange juice, from concentrate	1 cup	97

BEST SOURCES OF VITAMIN C *(continued)*

food	portion	vitamin C, mg.
papaya	1 medium	187
peas, green, raw	1/2 cup	31
sweet pepper, raw	1/2 cup	67
potato, baked with skin	1 medium	26
strawberries, fresh, sliced	1 cup	94
sweet potato, baked in skin, medium	1	28
tangerine, medium	1	26
tomatoes, ripe, raw	1 medium	23
vegetable juice cocktail	1 cup	67

VITAMIN C: A NATURAL ANTIHISTAMINE

Most people reach for the vitamin C at the first sniffle on the assumption that it will boost the immune system and shorten a cold's course. It seems that vitamin C can do that, but it may help more immediately by working as an antihistamine. Numerous studies have found that people taking various doses of vitamin C beyond the basic RDA suffered fewer attacks of bronchitis and asthma and a lower incidence of allergy symptoms. One thousand milligrams a day can soothe inflamed nasal passages and sinuses and ease congestion by reducing mucus production.

VITAMIN E: WHEN NATURAL IS BEST

In most cases, there is no reason to pay more for "natural" vitamin and mineral supplements. Vitamin E, however, is proving to be the exception. Although this fat-soluble antioxidant is present in many readily available vegetable oils, nuts, legumes, and grains, the concentration is low. You would have to eat massive amounts of these foods to obtain the 200 to 400 I.U.'s that studies have shown can do everything from reducing the risk of breast, prostate, and colorectal cancer to boosting the immune system and protecting the heart and arteries from the ravages of oxidation that lead to arteriosclerosis. Vitamin E can also reduce periodic breast tenderness and pain, and in massive doses, possibly slow the progress of Alzheimer's disease.

There are two different forms of vitamin E: synthetic and natural. While both have the same molecular structure, the differences between them are significant enough that our bodies retain twice as much natural E as synthetic. The recommendation: Get your vitamin E in its natural form. Read supplement labels and look for "d-alpha tocopherol," also known as "RRR-alpha." Avoid supplements made from "dl-alpha tocopherol" or "all-rac-alpha." Or, if you must take synthetic vitamin E, increase your dosage by one third to one half to compensate for what gets lost.

LEARN THE B, C, D'S OF BETTER BONES

There's a lot more to bones than just calcium, and a lot more to calcium than building good bones. But even if building bones was the only thing calcium did, this mineral would be worth more than its weight in gold. Calcium helps regulate cholesterol levels and heart function, lowers blood pressure, and plays a role in mood-affecting hormones. Calcium also stimulates enzymes that help us metabolize fat, may reduce the risk for colon cancer and cataracts, and helps prevent muscle cramps. Most important, though, calcium is the key ingredient in a diet-based plan to ward off future osteoporosis, the leading cause of disability in women. According to the National Institutes of Health, osteoporosis is among the four leading causes of death for women. One in five women who fracture a hip will die from the surgery to repair it or complications from the lengthy postoperative convalescence. And one in three women will fracture a hip by age eighty (compared to the approximately one in nine who develop breast cancer).

Knowing what we know, you'd think we couldn't get enough of it. And yet calcium deficiency is a major health problem. Experts estimate that fewer than 10 percent of women get all the calcium they need, and that up to 40 percent of us are deficient in vitamin D, which is crucial to calcium absorption. The problem is further complicated by the fact that we don't always absorb all the calcium we ingest, and even if we do, deficits in the crucial "helper" vitamins and minerals that support calcium can undermine our efforts. Every day most of us ingest too much of some common food or drink that either blocks our absorption of calcium or hastens its flushing from our systems.

Why You Need to Get Your Calcium Every Day

From the outside, our bones seem rock-solid, but, in fact, our bones are being built, broken down, and rebuilt every day. Osteoporosis occurs when the rate of rebuilding lags behind the rate of normal breakdown, leaving "holes" that weaken the bone and result in debilitating, even fatal, fractures. Our bodies use calcium for other functions, and the bones function as something of a calcium bank. When we fail to meet the calcium demand in other parts of our bodies, our cells start making "withdrawals." Without a bone-density test, you really have no idea what your "calcium balance" is.

We do most of our bone building by age thirty or so, and estrogen is crucial to the process. From early middle age on, the best we can do is preserve the bone we have and avoid further depletion. And lest anyone think that only women should be concerned with osteoporosis, men also lose bone density as they age, and can develop osteoporosis too.

HOW TO TAKE YOUR CALCIUM AND/OR CALCIUM SUPPLEMENTS

Do	Don't
Take your calcium with dairy foods or vitamin D.	Take your calcium with iron, iron-rich foods, or fiber, since each can block absorption.
Take several small doses a day, at least two hours before or after taking other mineral supplements.	Take calcium with other supplements except vitamin D.

HOW TO TAKE YOUR CALCIUM AND/OR
CALCIUM SUPPLEMENTS *(continued)*

Do	*Don't*
Avoid excessive protein (see "Protein: Pro and Con," page 131), caffeine (more than 3 cups of coffee or tea a day), fat (see "Fat: Unlocking the Right Combination," page 141), sodium (more than 2,400 mg. a day), phosphoric acid (found in diet sodas), and alcohol (more than two drinks a day), since they result in calcium being excreted.	Take supplements made from bone meal or dolomite; these may contain lead or arsenic.

THE RAW MATERIALS FOR BONES

WHAT YOU NEED EVERY DAY	WHAT IT DOES	WHERE TO GET IT
Boron • 2 mg.	Helps to slow calcium loss in women after menopause.	Legumes, green leafy vegetables, apples, pears, and grapes.
Calcium • 1,000 mg. all adults • 1,200 mg. adults over 50 • 1,500 mg. post-menopausal women	Calcium is essential to many crucial functions (see above).	Low-fat and nonfat dairy products (yogurt, skim milk), tofu, fish with bones (salmon, mackerel, sardines), bok choy, collard greens, kale, broccoli, and okra; supplements made with calcium citrate or calcium carbonate.

THE RAW MATERIALS FOR BONES *(continued)*

WHAT YOU NEED EVERY DAY	WHAT IT DOES	WHERE TO GET IT
Vitamin C • 60 mg.–200 mg.	An antioxidant, vitamin C increases calcium absorption. It is also a key component of collagen, which maintains and supports bones, teeth, and muscles.	Citrus fruit (oranges, grapefruit, etc.), cantaloupe, red peppers, and tomatoes.
Vitamin D • 400 I.U. up to age 51 • 600 I.U. over age 71	Vitamin D is crucial to calcium absorption and maintenance of blood calcium levels; in fact, deficiency in this vitamin has been pinpointed as a major factor in osteoporosis.	Vitamin D–fortified milk, eggs, salmon, sardines, eels, shrimp, chicken liver, pork liver. After just fifteen minutes of exposure to sunlight, your body synthesizes significant amounts of vitamin D.
Vitamin E • 300 I.U.	Vitamin E is an antioxidant that aids in healing.	Wheat germ, vegetable oils, whole-grain foods, liver, green leafy vegetables, dried beans, almonds, peanuts, cashews, soybeans, and sunflower seeds.
Magnesium • 280 mg.–400 mg.	Helps calcium bind to teeth and bones, among numerous other crucial functions.	Tofu, wheat germ, wheat bran, nuts, peanut butter, dried apricots, bulgur wheat, whole-wheat flour, fish, cereals, green vegetables, Swiss chard, spinach, bran, amaranth, broccoli, okra, pumpkin seeds, and squash seeds.

THE RAW MATERIALS FOR BONES *(continued)*

WHAT YOU NEED EVERY DAY	WHAT IT DOES	WHERE TO GET IT
Potassium • 200 mg.	Potassium is paired with calcium for a number of functions, such as regulating blood pressure. It is also an electrolyte. Legumes, green leafy vegetables, apples, pears, and grapes.	Nonfat dry milk, dried apricots, dried peaches, wheat germ, pumpkin seeds, squash seeds, almonds, peanuts, sardines, avocados, potatoes, dry lima beans, currants, raisins, turkey, pork, beet greens, spinach, and Swiss chard.

THE FACTS ABOUT NUTRITIONAL SUPPLEMENTS AND HERBAL REMEDIES

It's impossible to be a health-conscious consumer and not run headlong into a noisy parade of nutritional supplements—which may include vitamins, amino acids, botanical extracts, herbs, and other substances—that are the "next nutritional miracle." Selenium, chromium, amino acids, ephedra (ma huang), PC-SPES, royal jelly, feverfew, shark cartilage, yohimbe, ginseng, 5-HTP—the list goes on and on. And it will continue to as long as the regulatory agencies we trust to safeguard prescription and over-the-counter medications are denied jurisdiction over the unregulated, multibillion-dollar nutritional supplement industry.

Perhaps it's because we buy these products in the health food store, where everything is "natural" and "pure," but there's something about nutritional supplements that causes many of us to drop our guard. Imagine if someone handed you a box of a familiar over-the-counter antihistamine and said, "Well, this looks like the stuff you used to take, except the manufacturer hasn't had to do anything to ensure its purity. No agency can require him to make sure that every dose contains exactly the same concentration of active ingredients or require him to support this claim on the back that says it 'might prevent cancer.' " You'd probably refuse to take it, then demand that the

Food and Drug Administration pull the stuff off the market. Surprise! The FDA has virtually no authority over supplement manufacturers.

How big a problem this is was driven home in late 1998, when the *New England Journal of Medicine* published six papers detailing the dangers of unregulated dietary supplements. Incomplete or nonexistent labeling, wide variations in the content of active ingredients within the same product, and the undisclosed presence of dangerous ingredients (some intended, some not) were just a few of the dangers highlighted.

Among the findings:

- Two hundred sixty samples of herbal products imported from Asia were tested by the California Department of Health Services. Nearly one third of them—32 percent—also contained poisonous heavy metals such as arsenic, mercury, and lead.

- A patient who received zhong gan ling from her acupuncturist developed a condition in which all the body's white blood cells are eliminated. She had no way of knowing that the zhong gan ling also contained dipyrone, a drug banned in the United States because of its power to decimate white blood cells.

- Two women were hospitalized with irregular heartbeat, nausea, and vomiting after taking a "natural" preparation formulated to cleanse the digestive tract. Upon analysis, the preparation was found to be contaminated with digitalis—another natural drug derived from plants—an extremely potent heart drug that can bring on serious heart irregularities, even cardiac arrest, if taken improperly.

It's important to remember that the ingredients in supplements are potent medicine, with the same possible risks of any medicine but none of the safeguards now in place for government-regulated prescription and over-the-counter pharmaceutical products.

Here's how you can protect yourself:

- **KNOW EXACTLY WHAT YOU'RE TAKING.** Read the label and then research each ingredient for possible contraindications. Also be sure that you're getting the exact substance you want. Some herbal preparations, for instance, use different parts of the same plant, and these may have different effects. Also, learn and look for the Latin names of plants to be sure you're getting the right thing.

- **NO MATTER HOW PERSUASIVE THE LATEST STUDY, THE HEADLINE, OR THE SALES BROCHURE, DON'T RUSH OUT AND STOCK UP.** Historically, many groundbreaking studies don't bear up under careful scientific scrutiny, or their findings apply to a small segment of the population. Sometimes the results can't be duplicated, or the effect proves not to be as dramatic as first thought. Watch the news for a few months. Do your homework and give equal weight to experts who present a different opinion. As was the case with selenium, initial optimism often dims as new research and unforeseen side effects appear once millions of people try the new supplement.

- **NEVER INGEST MEGADOSES.** (See "Megadoses: Getting More—or Less—Than You Bargained For," page 193). Don't take megadoses without consulting a health professional, such as your doctor or a licensed dietician. There's still a lot we don't know about nutrition. For example, after decades of believing it is impossible to get too much vitamin C, scientists at the University of Leicester, England, discovered otherwise. In their study, this potent antioxidant actually fueled the free-radical activity it was supposed to slow in subjects who took 500 milligrams of vitamin C a day.

- **THINK LIKE A SCIENTIST.** When it comes to nutrition, we tend to think like this: "If a deficiency of Substance X causes muscle weakness, an excess of it will increase muscular strength." For better or worse, our bodies are much more complex than that. Any nutrient, no matter how "good," can have unexpected, serious, even fatal side effects when ingested in amounts much larger than what a normal, healthy diet provides.

- **DON'T BELIEVE THE HYPE.** Remember, nutritional-supplement manufacturers don't have to prove anything. While they must observe restrictions regarding what they print on a product's packaging and label, nothing stops them from making extravagant claims in brochures and handouts.

- **LEARN TO EVALUATE INFORMATION CRITICALLY.** Watch out for claims that include language such as "may . . . ," "have been shown to possibly . . . ," "are associated with . . . ," or "studies suggest that . . ."

- **IF YOU DO ADD NUTRITIONAL SUPPLEMENTS TO YOUR DIET, BUY ONLY PRODUCTS SOLD UNDER AN ESTABLISHED, WELL-KNOWN BRAND NAME.** Supplements are not inherently "safe." In 1989 thirty people died after taking

L-tryptophan—an amino acid then widely hailed as a "natural tranquilizer"— that had been contaminated. More recently, 5-HTP supplements, a related substance, were found to be contaminated.

ATHLETES AND DIETERS: THE BIGGEST TARGETS FOR QUESTIONABLE SUPPLEMENT CLAIMS

In health food stores and drugstores across the nation, all manner of supplements, powders, pills, and shakes that promise to improve athletic performance have taken over the shelves. People who are in less than optimal shape buy them too, hoping to jump-start their more modest fitness programs. Are these supplements worth it? Probably not.

In 1998, the President's Council on Physical Fitness and Sports issued a report on the efficacy of many nutritional supplements being promoted to improve physical performance, increase muscle mass, and reduce body-fat levels. The conclusion: There was "strong evidence" to support only caffeine, carbohydrates, water, creatine, and alkaline salts as substances that could enhance performance. Listed under the heading "weak evidence" were such widely touted supplements as amino acids, bee pollen, co-enzyme Q_{10}, conjugated linoleic acid (CLA), dehydroepiandrosterone (DHEA), ephedra (ma huang), ginseng, omega-3 fatty acids, protein, numerous vitamins and antioxidants, wheat germ oil, and yohimbe. The bottom line: ". . . Supplementation with various essential nutrients or commercial dietary supplements will NOT, in general, enhance exercise performance in well-nourished and physically active individuals."

MEGADOSES: GETTING MORE—OR LESS—THAN YOU BARGAINED FOR

Health-conscious people use the term *megadose,* but no one really knows what a megadose is. Experts loosely define a "megadose" as a daily intake that is at least triple or quadruple the RDA. The problem is that experts and researchers know much more about how our bodies respond to deficiencies than how they handle "overdoses." Despite this, there are many well known, influential doctors, researchers, teachers, and other experts who advise that we all take megadoses as a matter of course, whether they are indicated or not.

Much of the support for megadosing comes from studies that showed large doses of vitamins, minerals, and other supplements helped relieve specific conditions. It's important to remember that what may apply to the people in a given study may not apply to a normal, healthy person. If you do have a specific health concern and come across what you believe is compelling scientific research to support your taking megadoses, still proceed with caution. Learn the known side effects of high doses, and then discuss the matter with your physician or a health professional knowledgeable about nutrition (and that is not necessarily your workout instructor or the kid who stocks shelves at the health food store). Never take megadoses without your doctor's approval if you are pregnant, nursing, or taking a prescribed medication. Megadoses of some vitamins and minerals can interfere with the effectiveness of some medications and even "counteract" other nutrients.

For a long time, the common wisdom dictated concern only about the fat-soluble vitamins A, D, E, and K, because the body can accumulate and store up toxic levels. We know today that overdoses of water-soluble vitamins, including C and some of the Bs, can also create problems.

VITAMIN	RISKS OF MEGADOSING
Fat soluble	
A	*headache, liver damage, hair loss, blurred vision, skin rash, fatigue, nausea, diarrhea, jaundice, itchy eyes, dry skin, blood abnormalities, joint pain*
D	*irreversible kidney damage or heart damage, high blood pressure, weakened bones, nausea, kidney stones, high blood cholesterol*
E	*blurred vision, fatigue, upset stomach*
K	*has been shown to cause anemia in laboratory animals, but results are inconclusive*

VITAMIN	RISKS OF MEGADOSING *(continued)*
Water soluble	
B_1, *thiamine*	*not known, but there have been reports of headache, weakness, rapid heartbeat, insomnia, and fatigue*
B_3, *niacin*	*cramps, nausea, diarrhea, headache, jaundice, heartbeat irregularities, rash, liver damage, gout*
B_6, *pyridoxine*	*nerve damage that results in numbness and instability (usually reversible), insomnia, irritability, nervousness, increased urination (and bed wetting in children)*
C, ascorbic acid	*diarrhea, cramps, irritation of the urinary tract, kidney stones, bladder stones*

Getting Through the Day

6

Karen is in her early thirties, a pediatric emergency-room nurse and the single mother of a three-year-old boy. Although her mother and father live with her and she never has to worry about caring for her son, Karen still finds herself having a hard time making it through the day. The fact that she is sometimes assigned to different shifts or called in at the last minute to cover for a coworker also adds to her feeling that her life is getting out of control. She's read almost every health and fitness book out there, but she's lost patience with experts who presume their readers have time, resources, and options that simply don't exist in her life. Over the past two years, Karen has managed to lose 15 pounds and incorporate a few sessions of low-impact aerobics (done at home to a tape) and stretching into her weekly schedule. Since both of her parents suffer from high blood pressure, Karen is also interested in learning how to manage the stress in her life. As much as she would like to adopt a full fitness program, for now, she realizes that just getting through a tough day is her top priority.

BRAIN POWER AND BREAKFAST

It boosts your brain power, helps you concentrate, evens out your moods, and takes just fifteen minutes a day. What do we call this wondrous thing? Breakfast!

Breakfast breaks the fast (thus the name) we endure from the time we fall asleep until we wake up. In doing so, it raises our levels of glucose, a sugar that does for your brain what gasoline does for your car. Until recently, scientists have assumed that the brain receives a constant, steady supply of glucose independent of when and what kind of food was consumed throughout the day. Now we know that glucose levels fluctuate during the day and are lowest in the morning. And the brain has a ravenous appetite, claiming about 30 percent of your daily calories to keep working in top form. Failing to raise your glucose by eating has a direct effect on various brain functions, including the production of ACTH (adrenocorticotropic hormone), a pituitary hormone vital for memory, concentration, verbal skills, creativity, sociability, and physical performance. Skipping breakfast doesn't help you lose weight, either. In fact, skipping breakfast makes you more likely to eat throughout the day and eat more than you need.

To customize your own low-calorie (under 300), low-fat, high-fiber breakfast, simply choose one item from each of the three columns below. (Note: Even doubling up on one, two, or three items from each column would yield a 400-, 500-, or 600-calorie breakfast, which is also reasonable, depending on your requirements for the day.)

JOIN THE BREAKFAST CLUB

CARBOHYDRATE CHOICES	PROTEIN CHOICES	FRUIT AND VEGETABLE CHOICES
• 1 whole-grain waffle	• 2 egg whites, scrambled	• 3/4 cup orange juice
• 3/4 cup cooked farina or instant wheat cereal	• 1 poached or hard-boiled egg	• 1 medium apple or orange
• 2 slices light, whole-grain bread	• 1/2 cup plain, low-fat yogurt	• 1 small peach, pear, or nectarine
• 1/2 cup cooked oatmeal	• 1/2 cup low-fat (1%) cottage cheese	• 2 apricots
• 1/2 whole-wheat bagel	• 1 cup skim milk	• 1/2 medium banana
• 1 whole-wheat English muffin	• 1 tbsp. peanut butter	• tomato slices, mushrooms, peppers, onions
• 3/4 cup high-protein, low-fat cereal	• 1 oz. low-fat Swiss cheese	• 3/4 cup pineapple chunks in their own juice or fresh
		• 1/2 cup mixed berries or strawberries, blueberries, blackberries, or grapes
		• 1 cup cubed melon
		• 2 tbsp. spreadable fruit

THE CHEMISTRY BEHIND CRAVINGS—AND HOW TO BEAT IT

For many people a diet is a battleground, a moral war between the virtuous willpower and the evil craving. When our willpower prevails, we feel good about ourselves. When it fails, we mistakenly say that we have failed. But now we know that willpower isn't all it's cracked up to be, and that there's very little conscious will involved in avoiding cravings. They're real, and you can beat them, though not necessarily by simply trying to think your way around them.

Scientists aren't sure exactly what prompts food cravings, but they do know that up to 97 percent of all women experience them. While we tend to view a craving as a failure of willpower, circumstances beyond our conscious control are to blame, because when you satisfy a craving, you're doing more than just eating.

- **CRAVINGS ARE CHEMICAL.** They are the results of shifts in brain chemistry that are "corrected" by eating the desired food. It's not just coincidence that the foods we crave are usually carbohydrates, which elevate serotonin levels. When serotonin rises, it restores a general overall sense of well-being. (Interestingly, the most commonly craved food is chocolate, perhaps because it prompts the release of serotonin in the brain.)

- **THE FOODS WE CRAVE REMIND US OF SAFE, HAPPY TIMES.** Despite how our tastes change as we grow up, our childhood favorites never lose their power to comfort us. Perhaps it's the association with home, family, and Mom, or memories of being tucked in with a hot bowl of chicken noodle soup or a plate of cinnamon toast.

- **THE FOODS WE CRAVE NOT ONLY TASTE DELICIOUS, BUT FEEL GOOD.** The comfort foods we crave usually offer a multisensory experience. Creamy textures, for example, trigger the release of endorphins, brain chemicals that contribute to feelings of satisfaction and euphoria. Common comfort-food aromas—cinnamon, vanilla, and chocolate, for example—have been shown to increase sexual response, perhaps because they make us feel relaxed.

Cravings are not always diet busters, but a regular craving can undermine your healthy eating plan, depending on what it is you eat, how much, and how often. Since you can't banish cravings, here are some tips on how to handle them when they strike.

- **KEEP YOUR ENERGY UP, AND KEEP YOUR BLOOD SUGAR LEVEL.** Eat well-balanced meals throughout the day. Most of us experience a biologically induced drop in blood sugar in the late afternoon. A skimpy lunch will only exacerbate the drive to eat something to bring up energy.

- **DRINK PLENTY OF WATER.** And have as much of it iced as you like. Water fills your stomach, but an 8-ounce glass of ice water has the added advantage of forcing your body to burn calories to bring it up to body temperature.

- **THINK HOT TO THE TASTE AND HOT TO THE TOUCH.** To cool down your appetite, spicy foods such as horseradish, peppers, hot sauce, and hot salsa satisfy you quickly. Heated foods such as soup take longer to eat, so your brain gets a chance to signal that you're full before you've overeaten.

- **ANALYZE YOUR CRAVING BEFORE YOU TRY TO SATISFY IT.** What are you really hungry for? Try to discover what you really want instead of grabbing for anything handy. Then see if you can dissuade your craving by ignoring it temporarily. Take a walk, phone a friend, read that newspaper article you missed this morning. Chances are, the craving might disappear on its own.

- **IF YOU'RE DETERMINED TO SATISFY A CRAVING, DO IT AS SIMPLY AS POSSIBLE.** A craving for chocolate does not call for a half-pound box of chocolate-covered cherries; most of us can disarm the craving and pump up the serotonin with a Hershey's Kiss or two.

- **IT'S NOT NICE TO FOOL MOTHER NATURE.** Studies show that women who eat low-fat, low-calorie substitute foods often end up compensating by eating in quantity what they're not getting in quality. And remember, what you often crave in a craving is not simply the taste of chocolate, but the scent, the feel, even the look of it.

- **KEEP HEALTHY SUBSTITUTE MUNCHIES ON HAND.** Rice cakes, low-fat pretzels, air-popped popcorn, celery and carrot sticks, apple pieces, and banana chips are crunchy alternatives to more fattening chips and other mouth-pleasing crunchy snacks. However, if you notice that you grab a healthy munchy and then seek out the craved food as soon as you can, all you're doing is eating even more.

LOW BLOOD SUGAR: DO YOU HAVE IT?

must have low blood sugar!" How many times have you thought or heard this? Most of us associate feelings of exhaustion, inability to concentrate, and irritability with "low blood sugar," when in fact these really are typical symptoms of being hungry. This may indicate that your blood sugar at that point is at a low, but is not true hypoglycemia.

Normally, your body breaks down carbohydrates into a simple sugar called glucose, which enters the bloodstream. Insulin, a hormone produced by the pancreas, enables the glucose to move from the bloodstream to the cells, where it provides fuel. All of our cells need glucose, but the brain is particularly demanding and sensitive to dramatic fluctuations in glucose level. The healthy pancreas produces just the right amount of insulin to deliver the glucose to cells. Excess glucose is stored in the liver, so that the general blood-sugar level remains fairly consistent, between 70 and 120 for most adults.

When the blood sugar dips below 50, the condition is known as hypoglycemia, or low blood sugar. True hypoglycemia is rare among people who do not have diabetes, rare tumors, or conditions of the liver, kidneys, adrenal gland, or pituitary gland. People who consume excessive amounts of alcohol without eating and people who've undergone stomach surgery may also develop hypoglycemia. Some people experience what is called reactive hypoglycemia, which occurs when the blood "overreacts" to sugar intake, setting off a chain reaction in which blood sugar soars, insulin is dumped into the bloodstream, then the blood sugar drops dramatically. Adrenaline is produced, and prompts the liver to dump stored glucose into the bloodstream to protect the brain from a lack of sugar.

Why Is Hypoglycemia Over- and Underdiagnosed?

Because episodes of hypoglycemia have much in common with anxiety or panic attacks, doctors sometimes fail to distinguish between the two. In both, an adrenaline surge causes heart pounding, feelings of faintness and nervousness, sweating, and trembling. Even people with very vague symptoms that suggest anxiety are sometimes told they are hypoglycemic. It is also possible that some of us are just more sensitive to small fluctuations in blood sugar, even when they are in the normal range.

If You Think You Might Have Hypoglycemia

See your doctor if you experience the above symptoms, and don't settle for a diagnosis based solely on your description. You need a full, thorough workup that includes one or several oral glucose-tolerance tests given when you are experiencing symptoms. Only when low blood-sugar levels coincide with symptoms, and those symptoms are alleviated within fifteen minutes of eating, can a diagnosis of hypoglycemia be confirmed. If it is, then follow your doctor's advice on how to keep your blood-sugar levels stable throughout the day.

THERE IS A CURE FOR THE WINTERTIME BLUES

Where the holidays once kindled sweet memories, some of us now approach the season with a combination of dread and resignation. And with good reason, because staying fit and eating well are particularly challenging during the winter months—for some people, seemingly impossible. Why is that so?

- On average, we eat over 200 calories more a day in autumn and in winter than we do the rest of the year. The most obvious reason—or at least the one most of us prefer—is that it is a holiday season (one that kicks off with a night dedicated to gathering candy, no less). True, the traditional fare of Thanksgiving, Christmas, Hanukkah, New Year's Day, and other seasonal celebrations is usually rich in fat and calories.

- Daily cool-weather fare favors richer, calorie-dense foods at the same time that low-calorie alternatives—such as fresh fruits and vegetables—may be less easily available or less appetizing. And some people prefer to avoid fresh, out-of-season produce grown in foreign countries, where pesticide controls are lax or nonexistent.

- We tend to be less physically active in cold weather. Keeping to a regular exercise schedule takes a little more forethought and creativity. Your workout may seem more exhausting to you because, for example, you may not be drinking as much water now as you did in the summer. Remember: No matter what the temperature indoors or out, you need at least eight to ten glasses of water every day.

Could You Have Seasonal Affective Disorder (SAD)?

For over 15 million Americans, the wintertime blues are more than occasional, fleeting episodes of mild depression. First described in 1984, SAD is a form of seasonal depression whose symptoms include chronic fatigue, lethargy, sadness, sleep problems, difficulty concentrating, social withdrawal, and an increased craving for sweets and carbohydrates. Generally, SAD is a progressive disorder, meaning its symptoms grow more pronounced over time. Both men and women can experience SAD, but about 75 percent of the cases are women between the ages of twenty and fifty. The key hallmark of SAD is that it diminishes with the arrival of longer, warmer days in the spring. While no one is sure precisely what causes SAD, the connection between daily exposure to daylight and serotonin levels offers one answer. Serotonin generally falls a bit in the winter anyway. One theory is that people with SAD may have less serotonin to start with, and that the decreased exposure to daylight exacerbates the shortage.

Fortunately, there are simple things you can do yourself to offset the effects of SAD: exercise, manage stress, and get out into the daylight for a while each day. Light therapy is another effective treatment. This involves exposing yourself to special lights that encompass the full light spectrum, and mimic natural daylight and prompt serotonin production. If your depression is chronic and affecting your ability to function, consult a physician. Antidepressant medication is also effective in treating SAD.

WHY YOU MAY CRAVE MORE SWEETS IN THE WINTER

Researchers studying people with SAD made an interesting discovery that may shed light on why most of us find sweets and carbohydrates so irresistible in the colder months. In laboratory tests, people with SAD were asked to taste plain water, and water that had been flavored with sweet, sour, and bitter extracts. Compared to people who didn't have SAD, the test subjects could discriminate between one taste and another only when given water with much higher concentrations of flavoring. Interestingly, even the SAD sufferers who responded well to light therapy were still "taste blind." Researchers speculate that this diminished taste "sensation" may account for why people with SAD crave sugar- and fat-loaded foods, such as ice cream and chocolate: They deliver a stronger taste.

CAN YOU REALLY HOPE TO LOSE WEIGHT
DURING THE WINTER MONTHS?

Given what we know about metabolism and exercise habits, it's probably a little more difficult to stick to your health and fitness goals in the colder months. However, that doesn't mean it's impossible. By now, you probably have a good idea of what your particular cold-weather weak points are: the holiday meals, the temptation not to exercise, the impulse to "hibernate." Be realistic about where you've gotten into trouble in the past, and make reasonable plans to avoid those pitfalls this year.

If you suffer from seasonal affective disorder (SAD), you may opt to begin your new regimen once the weather warms up. In the meantime, you might try improving your lifestyle in a few specific areas, such as cutting down on fat or calories, learning healthier ways to cook, and beginning easy exercises that help you combat stress (see "Managing Stress," page 223). If you have had trouble sticking to a new eating or fitness plan in the past, or if you've just lost a substantial amount of weight, you might make your goal maintaining the weight you have now without losing or gaining any more.

WHAT YOUR SKIN MAY BE TRYING TO TELL YOU

If our eyes are windows to our souls, then our skin is a mirror of our overall health. Because skin is the largest, most visible organ we have, nutritional and health problems often show up there before we experience more severe symptoms. Your skin reveals a lot about your overall health, if you just know what to look for. Here's how your skin might be crying for help, and what you can do about it.

THE SKINNY ON THE SKIN YOU'RE IN

WHAT YOU SEE	WHAT IT SAYS	WHAT TO DO
Acne—50 percent of women between 20 and 50 develop adult acne.	You may be under stress.	Reevaluate the amount of rest and relaxation you get, as well as your diet. Be sure you're drinking enough water and eating a balanced diet.
	You may be experiencing a diminishing estrogen level.	Try over-the-counter remedies such as products containing benzoyl peroxide or alpha-hydroxy. Bear in mind that they can dry your skin. See your dermatologist or gynecologist about prescription topical treatments, antibiotics, or hormonal treatments.
	You may be washing your face too often or with cleansers that are too harsh for your skin and/or the season.	As we age, our skin gets drier. Most women find they have to alter their routine slightly in cold-weather months to make up for the lack of moisture in the air. Boost your intake of foods that contain vitamin A.
Blemishes, especially on your forehead and chin	You're eating too much fat, too much sugar, and too little fiber to help your body eliminate toxins and waste in a timely manner.	Cut the fat and the sugar, get 8 to 10 glasses of water every day, and increase your daily intake of fiber by eating more fresh fruits and vegetables. Also increase your intake of zinc through soybeans, oats, pumpkin and sunflower seeds, peanuts, pecans, pine nuts, whole-grain foods, oysters, and the dark meat of chicken.

THE SKINNY ON THE SKIN YOU'RE IN (continued)

WHAT YOU SEE	WHAT IT SAYS	WHAT TO DO
Chapped, dry lips	Either your lips aren't getting sufficient moisture to offset a dry environment (such as an office in winter) or you're not taking in enough fluid.	Protect and moisturize your lips as necessary. Make sure you're drinking 8 to 10 glasses of water every day.
Circles under the eyes	You may be stressed out, tired, and/or not eating or resting properly.	Get some more rest (yes, there is such a thing as a beauty sleep; see below) and eat a good, well-balanced diet.
Cold sores	These are caused by the herpes virus, which cannot be eliminated from the body. While the virus is always present, some people find that stress provokes an outbreak.	Increase your intake of vitamin C (see "Vitamin C: The First 'Superstar' Nutrient," page 182) and lysine, an amino acid found in dairy foods, eggs, legumes, and vegetables. Get more rest.
Dry skin around your lips, corners of your mouth, and nose that cracks	You may not be getting enough riboflavin, vitamin B_2, which is crucial to healthy red-blood-cell production.	If you drink a lot of caffeine or take certain types of prescription medications (namely, thyroid hormones, tricyclic antidepressants, and certain antipsychotics), your body may not be using all the B_2 you take in. Increase your intake of riboflavin through supplements, milk, almonds, wheat germ, yogurt, eggs, fortified cereals, cheese, pork, and liver.

THE SKINNY ON THE SKIN YOU'RE IN (continued)

WHAT YOU SEE	WHAT IT SAYS	WHAT TO DO
Exacerbation of existing skin conditions (such as eczema, hives, psoriasis, or acne)	You may be under intense emotional and/or physical stress that's drying your skin, increasing your level of androgen (a naturally occurring male hormone), and depleting your stores of vitamins A, B complex, C, and E.	Try to eliminate the source of stress. If you can't, get more rest and relaxation (including physical exercise), and increase your intake of vitamins A, B complex, C, and E. If symptoms persist or get worse, see a dermatologist.
"Flushed" rosy patches of skin (acne rosacea)	Your skin may be too dry, you may be overstressed, or you may be drinking too much alcohol.	Eliminate possible causes. Moisturize, drink plenty of water, reduce stress, and cut down on or eliminate alcoholic beverages. If this does not help, see your dermatologist, who can prescribe treatment.

SLEEP YOUR WAY TO BEAUTY

It sounds too good to be true. All those jokes we made about "getting our beauty sleep" weren't so silly after all. Scientific studies now confirm what most of us always wished were true: Sleep is essential to beautiful skin. The pituitary gland secretes growth hormone, which is responsible for the cell regeneration essential for glowing, supple skin. Apparently, our bodies are too "preoccupied" when we're awake and active to work on cell regeneration and repair. This activity increases by 300 percent when we're sleeping, peaking at 1:00 A.M. (but only if you're sleeping then). At around the same time, estrogen and progesterone—two hormones crucial to healthy skin—are also peaking. Good night!

SAVE FACE: THE MUSCLES YOU SHOULD NEVER EXERCISE

We've all seen the infomercials, magazine articles, ads, and books trumpeting the new way to keep your face smooth, youthful, and face-lift-free: the so-called facial workout. The basic premise—that you can firm your cheeks, chin, and forehead by exercising the muscles in your face (some programs even involve miniature exercise equipment that fits inside your mouth or under your chin)—sounds logical, but it's a terrible idea. Working out your face does not improve your looks. If anything, it does precisely the opposite. Why?

The three leading causes of wrinkles are sun damage, aging, and normal facial movement. The basic premise of facial workouts ignores the role of facial movement in creating wrinkles, and states, erroneously, that wrinkles and sagging are due to a loss of muscle tone. In fact, the real culprits are the natural deterioration and breakdown of the skin and the fat beneath it. And think about it: Your facial muscles get a good workout every time you smile, chew, laugh, or frown. Ironically, one of the latest treatments for wrinkles, injections of weakened botulism toxin, has a smoothing effect because the toxin essentially paralyzes targeted facial muscles, causing them not to move.

Facial muscles are unique among muscles in that they attach directly to the skin, not to surrounding bone. The muscles on the forehead, around the eyes, and around the mouth can be strengthened, but the result will not be what you had in mind. When you make these muscles stronger, you increase their pull on the skin they attach to, and the result is deeper lines.

IT'S ALL IN THE TIMING

Daily and monthly biological cycles present us with opportunities to use our time more effectively and get the most benefit out of anything we do, from exercising to undergoing routine medical tests.

Your Daily Clock

- **BLOOD SUGAR LEVEL—AND THE ABILITY TO CONCENTRATE AND FOCUS CLEARLY**—is at its lowest ebb first thing in the morning.

- **CREATIVITY** is at its highest between roughly 9:00 A.M. and 10:00 A.M. Use this time to brainstorm and write.

- **ALERTNESS** is highest right before noon, which makes this prime time for dealing with matters that require logic.

- **MEMORY** works best in late afternoon or early evening. You are more likely to retain what you've learned then than if you'd stayed up late to cram.

- **SLEEPINESS** comes over most of us in the afternoon between 1:00 P.M. and 4:00 P.M. and in the early morning hours after 2:00 A.M. and before 6:00 A.M. If possible, catching even a brief catnap in the late afternoon will help you stay focused and energized for the rest of the day.

- **SEVERAL PHYSICAL ABILITIES RELATED TO EXERCISE PERFORMANCE— FLEXIBILITY, REACTION TIME, COORDINATION, STRENGTH, AND AEROBIC CAPACITY**—are at their highest between 4:00 P.M. and 7:00 P.M.

The Monthly Calendar (For Women Only)

The secret to staying healthy and looking great may lie in your calendar. That's because fluctuations in hormone levels may make you more sensitive to pain or discomfort or cause physical changes that can affect medical diagnosis and treatment.

- Two weeks before your period is the best time to donate blood (but only if you're not anemic). It's probably a good time to take a long weekend away with your mate, since sexual desire coincides with ovulation.

- One week before your period is the best time to get a massage, or do anything for yourself that makes you feel good and a little bit pampered, or see your dermatologist or gynecologist for a standard checkup.

- The week after your period is the best time for waxing, electrolysis, dental work, and undergoing chemical facial peel and diagnostic tests that involve radiation (X rays, mammograms, etc.). These procedures will all be less uncomfortable because your body isn't retaining preperiod water. It's also the best time to start a new way of eating, since food cravings will be at their lowest point, and an exercise program, since you'll feel lighter and more energized.

THREE EASY EXERCISES TO REPLENISH YOU

The Stimulating Breath

For times that call for a quick pick-me-up—when you get a little drowsy behind the wheel or feel that mid-afternoon slump at your desk—here's a yogic exercise that works faster than a cup of coffee. Commonly known as the "bellows breath," it's also called the stimulating breath. The first time you try this exercise, keep it up for no longer than fifteen seconds, then breathe normally. Each time you do it, increase the duration by increments of five seconds, if you can, until you work up to a full minute.

Try doing it every morning when you first get up. This is real exercise, so expect to feel some fatigue in the muscles you are using at first. You should feel significantly more alert, an effect that will increase with practice.

1. Sit with your back straight and put your tongue in the yogic position, as described on page 21. Hold it there for the duration of the exercise.

2. Inhale and exhale very rapidly through your nose, keeping your mouth tightly closed. Your inhalations and exhalations should be of equal length and as short as possible, and you should do them as fast as possible. You should feel muscular effort at the base of your neck just above the collarbone and at your diaphragm (place your hands on these spots to feel the movement). The action of your chest should be rapid and mechanical, like a bellows pumping air.

3. Resume normal breathing.

The Ultimate Three-Minute Oxygen Booster

Anytime is a good time to boost your energy, creativity, focus, and inspiration. Try this:

1. Sit with your arms stretched out to your sides, at shoulder level.

2. Bring your arms up over your head, so that your wrists cross.

3. Begin breathing for ultimate oxygenation: through your nose only. This forces you to take deeper breaths. Breathe with your whole chest and stomach. Stay focused.

Total Body Tension Tamer/Energizer

You are exhausted, barely able to keep your eyes open—and it's only two in the afternoon. Don't fight it. Remember, when your eyes are tired, everything is tired. Times like this, a nap would be ideal, but for most of us, that's unrealistic. Try the following nap-replacing energizer:

1. At a table (or desk), sit with your feet flat on the floor and rest your elbows on the table. It's important to keep your head up and your spine straight, so if necessary, place a pillow, books, or a stack of papers under your elbows.

2. Rub your palms together until they feel warm, then bring them to your eyes, but don't touch your eyes. Keep your fingers interlocked just above the bridge of your nose.

3. Close your eyes and breathe deeply and rhythmically (see "Take a Real Breather," page 21). Imagine the air circulating behind your eyes and carrying away with it all the tension in your body.

4. Continue breathing this way until you feel refreshed. Or until someone taps you on the shoulder and tells you to get back to work!

WORKING LATE? GAINING WEIGHT? HERE'S WHY

Burning the midnight oil to meet that deadline or to straighten up the house may be doing more to damage your health than just depriving your body of sleep. New research confirms what many of us already know: A lack of sleep results in increased appetite, increased eating, and increased weight. The question is, Why?

It's the Rhythm of Life

Try as you might, you'll probably never be able to fully reset or override the body clock of your circadian rhythms. Most adults need eight hours of sleep every night to function at their best. Any disruption in normal sleeping-waking patterns can result in an increased appetite. This explains why when you're suffering from jet lag, you might feel especially hungry. People who work nights or alternate between working day shifts and night shifts tend to overeat. One possible reason is that good, healthy meals may not be as readily available during their work time. It also seems that we not only eat more at night but are less discriminating about what and how much we eat.

As far as your body is concerned, nighttime is the right time for sleeping. Your brain produces neurochemicals that set the stage for the nightly fast that accompanies it. In other words, your metabolism slows to "save up" energy between nighttime and breakfast. The result is that your body temperature drops and you burn fewer calories than you would in the daytime.

Nighttime Cravings

When you stay up late, you encounter biologically induced cravings you would miss if you were asleep:

- **FAT.** The neurochemical galanin creates our appetite for fat and helps determine how our bodies store it. Galanin levels change throughout the day, from a morning low to a late-night peak, which may explain why ice cream, potato chips, and chocolate are favorite late-night snacks.

- **CARBOHYDRATES.** If you're up late at night, your body is probably producing extra cortisol, a hormone the body produces in response to fatigue and stress. Cortisol tends to make us feel anxious. Once we ingest carbohydrate-rich foods, the body then has the raw materials it needs to produce serotonin, the neurochemical that calms us and counteracts the effects of cortisol. Cortisol can rise at any time during the day, but we are more likely to be tired and overwhelmed at night, especially if we have to stay awake too long to perform complex, challenging work.

- **SUGAR.** Staying up late can induce sugar cravings two ways. Declining blood-sugar levels signal your body to eat, and being tired often prompts us to grab for high-sugar foods to perk us back up.

- **FOOD IN GENERAL.** When you are consistently sleep-deprived, your basic body temperature drops, and your appetite increases to provide the calories to bring your body temperature back up to normal. Research on sleep-deprived rats found that body temperature consistently declined even when they consumed enough calories to raise it.

Six Night Owl Tips

If you must stay up late or get by with less sleep than you need, there are ways to out-smart your body and avoid putting on those nighttime pounds.

1. **KEEP YOUR FOOD INTAKE CONSISTENT AND ADEQUATE THROUGHOUT THE DAY.** This is true for every day, but especially if you're expecting a long night ahead. Be sure you have a good lunch, an afternoon snack, a good dinner, and a healthy snack sometime between dinner and late night.

2. **DON'T COME HOME HUNGRY.** Right before you leave work or on the way home, try a light, carb-rich snack: some low-fat pretzels, rice cakes, an English muffin, air-popped popcorn, an apple, or almonds. It will keep your blood-sugar level steady and short-circuit a feeding frenzy.

3. **IF YOU'RE STRESSED OUT, RECOGNIZE THAT YOU ARE RESPONDING WITH FOOD AND CHOOSE THE RIGHT FOOD SOOTHER.** We all know the feeling: You walk in the door, head straight for the kitchen, and grab the first thing you see—anything to give you a lift. You know it's only thirty minutes to dinnertime, but you can't resist that fourth Oreo or second slice of cheese. Stop! Be sure you have on hand—and highly visible—healthy alternatives that are small, soothing, and carbohydrate-rich: a banana, grapes, yogurt, low-fat chocolate milk, a veggie quesadilla, or baby carrots.

4. **PICK YOURSELF UP WITH SOMETHING OTHER THAN FOOD.** If it's possible to plan your late night, try: grabbing a twenty-minute nap after dinner; taking a quick shower (if possible use bath products with invigorating scents, such as rosemary, eucalyptus, citrus, or peppermint); exercising for ten or fifteen minutes; drinking one or more tall glasses of ice water; dancing to a few songs; brushing your teeth; washing your face with cool water; breathing fresh air; phoning a friend; taking care of your houseplants; playing with your pet; giving yourself a facial or conditioning your hair; meditating; reading the next chapter of a book; writing a letter to a friend; or indulging in your hobby (gardening, playing an instrument, painting, sewing, etc.).

5. **DON'T FORGET CAFFEINE.** True, caffeine is not for everyone, and you should avoid it if it's going to keep you up even after you've finished your late-night work. However, caffeine has near-miraculous powers to keep you awake (it blocks adenosine, a neurochemical that lets you know you're tired) and to help you focus your attention on the task at hand.

6. **IF YOU MUST BE A NIGHT OWL, SNACK WISELY.** Face it: Staying up late or drastically altering your established biological rhythms will produce biochemical changes that include hunger and a weakened ability to eat sensibly. Instead of beating yourself up because you're snacking at 2:00 A.M., be sure you have the right snacks on hand.

DOES IT MATTER WHEN I EAT DINNER?

Yes. Even though only a few hours separate 6:00 P.M. from 10:00 P.M., your body responds to the calories you take in very differently. The later you eat, the more slowly your body will metabolize calories. This is because it's helping "save up" for the overnight fast ahead. Another reason you may opt for the earlier dinnertime is that eating late means you'll probably awaken with a high blood-sugar level and not feel hungry enough to eat breakfast—the most important meal of the day. People who eat most of their calories in the evening tend to skip breakfast, kicking off a domino effect of poor eating habits through the rest of the day: the mid-morning donut, the high-fat lunch, the constant noshing, and the big dinner—usually with some snacking before and after.

THE SEVEN BEST LATE-NIGHT SNACKS

Remember: Carbohydrates tend to make you sleepier. Protein metabolizes more steadily, to produce a steady blood-sugar level. And sugar is probably what you crave the most. Here are seven healthy ways to satisfy your nighttime cravings and give your brain what it needs to keep going.

1. Low-fat yogurt; fruit-flavored varieties that include sugar will give you a little extra boost
2. Lean chicken, fish, or meat
3. Seeds and nuts
4. Cheese
5. Eggs
6. Tofu
7. Beans

HAVE A TRULY GOOD NIGHT: LEARN TO SLEEP

Most of us accept our restless or sleepless nights as the normal consequence of our busy lives. We shouldn't. Sleep is something we're born knowing how to do but over time seem to forget. By the time we reach adulthood, our sleep begins to diminish in both quality and quantity. In fact, leading sleep experts warn that we are a nation in the midst of a sleep deprivation epidemic of alarming proportions. How bad is it? The National Traffic Safety Administration claims that 100,000 accidents, 1,500 deaths, and 71,000 injuries are due to drivers who don't get enough sleep. More than half of Americans have trouble sleeping; one third of those surveyed recently claimed to sleep six hours or less a night during the workweek. Sleep problems affect how well we function, how good we feel, and even how we look. There's no question about it: Lack of sleep stresses our bodies and our minds.

How little sleep is too little? Just getting a half hour less than you need a night has been shown to have a negative impact on mental performance and attitude. Judgment, attention, and short-term memory are all affected by getting less than optimal sleep. Missing a few hours' sleep a week will compromise your exercise performance and make it difficult to stick to new eating habits, too. And contrary to popular belief, you cannot "make up" the sleep you missed by rising late on your days off. Better to get up at your normal time and accomplish the tasks that keep you up late during the week so you can retire earlier.

Sleep is more than simply rest. In fact, it is while we are sleeping that many biological processes go into full gear. It is only in the deepest sleep that the pituitary gland releases HGH, the growth hormone that prompts cells to divide and replace old ones. In children and young people, this results in growth. In older people, it's basically a repair-and-maintenance operation that keeps us looking and feeling our best. As we age, our production of HGH declines, in large part because we don't sleep enough to allow optimum HGH release.

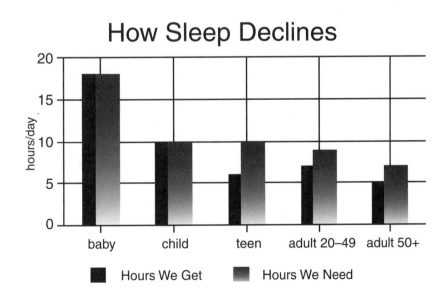

How Sleep Declines

- **RECOGNIZE THE SIGNS OF SLEEP DEPRIVATION.** If you find yourself dozing off at the movies, in the theater, while watching television, reading a book, or listening to someone speak, you are sleep deprived. Most of us just assume that these are signs of boredom, but boredom doesn't make your eyelids drop—sleeplessness does.

- **HAVE A CALMING BEDTIME ROUTINE.** Wind down from your day. Use the hours before bedtime to slow down and relax. Meditate, exercise (if it doesn't keep you awake), write in your journal, read a book, watch television, play with your children—whatever makes you feel calm.

- **DON'T LET YOUR DIET KEEP YOU AWAKE.** Alcohol, caffeine, and nicotine can keep you awake; avoid them after late afternoon or eliminate them entirely. If indigestion is keeping you awake, identify the problem (lactose intolerance, spicy food, too much fat, meals that are too large) and correct it.

- **EAT YOUR WAY TO BETTER SLEEP.** Foods that contain an amino acid called L-tryptophan, which has a calming, sedating effect, might help. Turkey, chicken, tuna, milk, and eggs are all rich in L-tryptophan. Calming herbal teas, such as chamomile and valerian, might also help.

- **MAKE YOUR BEDROOM YOUR SLEEP ROOM.** The room you spend a third of your life in should be special. Years ago, bedrooms were sleep sanctuaries that had one purpose: promoting good sleep (well, if you count sex, two). Today the bedroom has become a combination office, playroom, snack table, and family home theater. The mere presence of televisions and VCRs encourages late-night viewing, for example. Keep your bedroom on the cool side, around 65 degrees F, with plenty of fresh air.

- **TRY A HOT SHOWER OR HOT BATH.** Raising your body temperature relaxes your muscles and makes you feel sleepier. One study found that women who took a hot shower two hours before they went to sleep woke up less frequently in the night and experienced twenty minutes more deep sleep.

- **PUT YOURSELF ON A SLEEP SCHEDULE.** When do you feel sleepy? That's when you should go to bed. Not "after the eleven o'clock news," "after Letterman," or "after I finish this chapter." The moment you feel tired, hit the hay. Try to stick to your schedule through holidays and weekends, too. While it's okay to sleep in now and then, finding and sticking to a sleep schedule is the best way to improve your sleep.

- **JUST DO IT.** Easier said than done for some of us, perhaps, but whenever possible heed the call to sleep, even for fifteen or twenty minutes. It's a well-known fact that we get sleepy between 1:00 P.M. and 4:00 P.M. and between 2:00 A.M. and 6:00 A.M. If possible, put your head down on your desk for fifteen minutes or grab a quick catnap. In the long run, you'll be more refreshed than if you'd had that cup of coffee.

- **EXERCISE REGULARLY.** People who make exercise part of their lives sleep better. Some people can exercise within a few hours of bedtime and sleep like babies; others find the stimulation keeps them up.

- **CONSULT YOUR DOCTOR OR SEE A SLEEP SPECIALIST IF YOU EXPERIENCE ANY OF THE FOLLOWING SYMPTOMS:**

  restless legs syndrome, an unpleasant sensation in the calf muscles that makes you
      feel as though you must move your legs;
  loud snoring;
  insomnia;
  sleep apnea, a potentially life-threatening condition in which breathing ceases
      from several to hundreds of times a night;
  chronic exhaustion;
  waking up feeling as though you've been dreaming most of the night;
  chronic irritability;
  trouble falling asleep within thirty minutes of going to bed;
  difficulty relaxing because you can't stop thinking or worrying;
  problems falling back to sleep once you've awakened.

THE BIOCHEMICAL WONDER OF A HOT BATH

We all know a hot bath can make us drowsy, but how does it work? If you assumed it had something to do with relaxing muscles, you're only partially right. Every evening, in response to our circadian rhythms, our core body temperature gradually begins dropping. This drop is what makes us feel sleepy. You emerge from your hot bath with an elevated body temperature, which your body then lowers. The significant drop in temperature is what induces sleep.

BREATHE EASIER AT NIGHT

Dust mites—microscopic insects that are ubiquitous and nestle invisibly in mattresses, pillows, and bedclothes—may be the cause of your sinus problems, sore throat, runny nose, or asthma attacks. Considering we spend about a third of our lives in bed, it's a good idea to make the air we breathe there as clean as possible. While you may not totally eradicate dust mites, you can reduce their numbers significantly by covering your mattresses and pillows in mite-proof sheets or plastic covers and washing your bedding once a week in very hot water. Adding a bit of eucalyptus oil to the wash water will give your linens an invigorating scent and deters the little buggers. You might also consider purchasing a HEPA-quality air purifier, which can remove up to 99 percent of dust and other allergens from the air.

DROWSY AT YOUR DESK? GETTING THROUGH THE MORNING AFTER

Here are some tips to get you through those mornings when your desk blotter or mouse pad starts to look as inviting as your pillow:

- **STICK TO THE KINDS OF TASKS YOU CAN DO EASILY NOW.** Exhaustion takes its toll first on creative thinking, cognitive functioning, and self-control. This may not be the best day to balance the company checking account or discuss with your boss why you shouldn't have been passed over for that promotion. If you can, avoid anything that involves planning, thinking on your feet, or sensitive discussions or confrontations until you're better rested.

- **WHAT TO CONCENTRATE ON WHEN YOU CAN'T.** Now's a good time to file those papers, collect your expenses receipts, treat your assistant to lunch, or organize your bookshelves.

- **KEEP MOVING.** Take the long way around to a colleague's office, pick up your own copying, or circle the block on your lunch hour. Anything that boosts your circulation and increases oxygen flow to the brain will help you focus better.

- **SHIFT GEARS.** Try not to stick to any one task for too long. Alternate your activities, even if it means breaking up three or four tasks into half-hour bits.

- **RESIST CAFFEINE TEMPTATION.** While one jolt of caffeine can give you a boost, too much more and the law of diminishing returns goes into effect. Three or four cups of coffee, researchers have found, can actually precipitate an energy slump.

- **EAT CAREFULLY.** Be sure your lunch provides: 50 percent of calories from carbohydrates, 30 percent from protein, and 20 percent from fat. Today is not the day to stick to a crash or extremely low fat, low-carb plan.

- **NAP FOR FIFTEEN MINUTES.** And if you can't do that, at least breathe. (See "Take a Real Breather," page 21.)

A HANGOVER CURE

This is a good drink for that morning after overindulging in alcohol. Not only will it replenish the fluids the alcohol sapped, but it's rich in vitamins and minerals, and the vegetables and spices are also good for detoxing. Bottoms up!

In a blender combine and blend until smooth:

4 cups vegetable juice, preferably spicy
2 stalks celery, coarsely chopped
1 bunch fresh parsley, coarsely chopped
1 1/2 cups water
1 cup chopped onions
2 tablespoons chopped fresh basil *or* 2 teaspoons dried
2 teaspoons hot pepper sauce
1 teaspoon rosemary leaves

Once you've blended all the ingredients, pour into a large pot and bring to a boil. Lower the heat and simmer for 30 minutes. Drink hot or cold.

STRETCH YOUR WAY THROUGH THE STRETCH

We know that nothing feels better than a good stretch, so why don't we do it more often? A deep stretch can be both relaxing and revitalizing—the perfect combination to get you through those slump times, such as those late afternoons at your desk or that hour right before you start cooking dinner. Here's a yogic exercise to stretch away all the tension you've built up through the day.

1. Sit up in your chair with your back straight.

2. Take a deep breath and focus on where your shoulders are. Without making a jerking motion or shrugging hard, gently lower them.

3. Stretch your right arm straight up over your head, then bend your elbow, and bring your hand down so that your palm touches your back between your shoulder blades.

4. Stretch your left arm behind you, so that your left hand is against your middle back, just above your waistline, with your hand pointing up and your palm facing away from your body.

5. If you can, clasp your hands. If you can't reach comfortably, use a small towel, a sock, or something else to bridge the gap. Place it in your right hand and grasp it with your left.

6. Stretch up through your right elbow while at the same time stretching down through your left elbow. Don't jerk; this should be a slow, subtle movement.

7. Hold the stretch for twenty seconds while breathing normally; repeat on the other side.

BECOME MORE MENTALLY AND PHYSICALLY ALERT IN TEN MINUTES

We sit at work, sit in our cars, sit at home, and then find ourselves vegging out in front of the television, the computer, or the big box of cookies because we just can't summon the energy to do anything else. The obvious answer to counteracting the effects of inactivity is to be active, but we don't seem inclined to do that. We feel so drained, we go for the quickest energy jolt we can get for the least amount of physical effort.

There's only one way to get the energy you need to move, and that's to move. A recent study showed that a brisk ten-minute walk restored energy far more reliably and effectively than a sugar fix. The results were longer lasting too. Ten minutes of walking—indoors or out—increased both mental and physical alertness for an hour or more. And that ten-minute jaunt will burn off about 50 to 70 calories and raise your metabolism, so you are less likely to snack.

WHAT'S GREAT ABOUT THE GREAT OUTDOORS

In addition to getting some fresh air, you can also grab some mood-enhancing rays. Researchers at Boston University found evidence to suggest that exposure to sunlight prompts the skin to produce beta-endorphins, even when you're wearing sunscreen. And if you spend just fifteen minutes in the sun each day—which experts consider safe in terms of skin cancer risk—you may reduce your risk of developing breast cancer by 40 percent. We know that vitamin D, produced by the skin in the presence of ultraviolet rays, has an anticancer effect if taken as a supplement of 200 I.U. or more daily.

MANAGING STRESS

Stress. We hear the word all the time, and most people would say they live with stress every day. All too often, the best-laid eating and exercise plans are undermined by the stress we experience in our daily lives. Whether the stress is short term (such as getting stuck in traffic on your way to an important meeting) or long term (such as caring for a chronically ill family member), our bodies respond to stress with neuro-chemicals that make it more difficult for us to care for ourselves as we should.

What Does Stress Do?

When we're confronted with stressful situations, our brains respond by releasing "stress hormones," adrenaline and cortisol, in preparation to flee or fight. That's why your heart rate and respiration increase, your blood pressure soars, and your muscles tighten. On a deeper chemical level, adrenaline and cortisol have other lasting effects. High rates of cortisol have been shown to hinder memory in rats. When adrenaline prepares your body to face a threat, it signals a precipitous rise in blood sugar to meet the anticipated demand from muscles tensed for action. Since in real life we are rarely in situations from which we must literally run for our lives or physically defend ourselves, this "readiness" results in tension and anxiety. It's as if our bodies were all dressed up—to fight—with no place to go.

Repeated surges in cortisol have been known to suppress the immune system, making it easier for infection to take hold. In women cortisol has been shown to prompt a craving for sweet and high-fat foods. Stress also causes a drop in serotonin levels, and interestingly, women's serotonin levels drop more quickly than men's and take longer to recover. Low serotonin levels prompt a craving for carbohydrates. Put these cravings together, and it's easy to see why a piece of chocolate cake or a pint of Ben & Jerry's looks so good when we're stressed out. Unfortunately, stress can make us susceptible to even more damaging indulgences. When we experience more physiological stress than our bodies can resolve, we try to relax and unwind by not only excessive eating, but drinking, smoking, and using illegal drugs. Of course, these destressors work only temporarily, and then we're hooked back into the same cycle again.

Breaking the Stress Cycle

First, realize that stress sets off chemical and physiological changes that may be beyond your control. To many of us, stress-provoking situations are foreseeable. And before you say, "I don't have time to help myself deal with stress," remember that having poor eating habits and failing to exercise regularly are in and of themselves causes of stress. If you anticipate or find yourself in a stress period, try the following:

- **PLAN TO EAT RIGHT ALL DAY THROUGH.** By now you probably know what foods you'll be tempted to reach for. Eliminate them from your desk, your pantry, and your briefcase now. Instead, be sure you have "planted" the healthy, complex-carbohydrate-rich alternatives: unsalted almonds, bananas, dried apricots, raisins, oranges, grapefruit, yogurt, rice cakes, bagels, strawberries, legumes, and sweet potatoes.

- **EAT ON A STRESS SCHEDULE.** That means opt for smaller, more frequent meals throughout the day or three large meals with strategic snacking in between. This keeps your blood sugar up and level.

- **IF YOU DON'T EAT RIGHT, SUPPLEMENT FOR STRESS.** Stress depletes your body of important nutrients. Try to be sure you get enough vitamin C, magnesium, vitamin A, and vitamin B complex (especially B_{12}, which is harder to get through diet).

- **DRINK ENOUGH WATER.** Eight to ten glasses a day, *minimum*. Be especially mindful about resorting to "water substitutes" such as soft drinks, caffeinated beverages, and juice and sports drinks that are high in sugar. These will either dehydrate you or send your blood sugar soaring.

- **MAKE TIME TO EXERCISE.** Nothing does more to turn back the physical effects of stress than exercise. Simply taking a half hour or so to yourself—whether you spend it doing tai chi, breathing exercises, or taking a brisk walk—will help tremendously. Physical exercise produces countless positive effects, such as giving you more energy and facilitating better sleep, that counteract the ravages of stress. Skip the punching bag, though. Recent research finds that acting out aggressively increases rather than decreases anger.

- **LET THE SUNSHINE IN.** When you're exposed to sunlight, your brain produces more serotonin. Just fifteen minutes a day will not only brighten your mood but will increase your level of vitamin D.

STRESS, EXERCISE, AND YOUR IMMUNE SYSTEM

Exercise can help relieve the physiological changes stress induces, and pump up the immune system, which protects our bodies from all manner of infections and dispatches millions of cancer cells before they take hold and multiply into tumors.

So if a little exercise is good for you, a lot must be better, right? Wrong. While moderate exercise benefits the immune system, strenuous exercise—which is any form of activity that you cannot do with reasonable ease—is a form of stress itself.

Of course, true athletes feel compelled to push beyond their limits and improve performance, which is fine as long as you're healthy. If, however, you sweat profusely, find it difficult to talk while you're working out, feel notably more fatigued than usual afterward, experience unsteadiness, or have muscle pain that is pronounced and/or chronic, you may not only be overdoing it, you may be doing yourself more harm than good. Surprisingly, researchers have found that athletes who train very hard are actually more—not less—likely to develop disease. And if your body is fighting any infection more serious than a mild cold—that is, any kind of infection, influenza, pneumonia, or bronchitis—take a rest from your workout. Rather than bolster your immune system, your workout will only be diverting the energy your body needs to overcome the infection and heal.

TURN IT DOWN

Most people know that extremely loud noise can be harmful to our hearing, but we don't always recognize the role noise plays in creating stress. Loud noise is an obvious offender. Ninety decibels (dBs) is considered potentially detrimental to hearing, and we are exposed to that level several times a day, from piercing car alarms, sirens, loud radios, and other noises of daily life. But these are not nearly as stressful as the everyday noise we probably think we ignore. Some surprising culprits: crying babies, overamped sound systems in movie theaters and concert halls, and vacuum cleaners. And don't overlook your health club. One study found that almost 60 percent of health clubs that used music were playing it above 100 dBs.

At the other end of the noise spectrum are sounds that we don't necessarily perceive as loud but that can induce stress nonetheless. Try a few days of turning off the TV or radio unless you're actively listening and see how much more relaxing it is when everyone in the house isn't trying to talk over some other background noise. Become aware of the "light buzz" emanating from computer equipment, printers, typewriters, and other office machines, as well as from air conditioners, air purifiers, and humidifiers. If you're feeling particularly stressed, try to remove at least some of the noise for a set period each day.

SLEEP, COLD WATER, AND CLEAR THINKING

Does stress or worry ever keep you from sleep? Do you ever lie in bed, wide awake, thinking and rethinking the same problem through, with no end in sight? If so, you might take some old advice—sleep on it—with a new, refreshing twist.

There is some scientific evidence to support the idea of sleeping on a problem. According to Dr. Arthur White, of the SpineCare Medical Group, in San Francisco, while you're sleeping, your right brain dominates, presenting patterns, possibilities, and solutions the conscious left brain might not have produced or might have rejected. Our sleeping brains probably do a lot more problem-solving work than we know. We all know the experience of having a vivid dream that we are utterly unable to recall upon waking. It seems to be a similar situation with right-brain nighttime problem solving, but there's something you can do. Upon waking, take a sip of cold water, then state the problem aloud in clear, simple language. Repeat it several times over a few minutes. Chances are, the combination of cold water and the verbal prompts will reactivate your right brain and bring its solution from the back of your mind to the tip of your tongue.

Getting the Edge

7.

. . . .

Simone and Paul are a married couple in their early fifties. Always health conscious, they first came to me a couple of years ago after Paul's father passed away. Like so many people their age, Simone and Paul were caught between two generations of family who needed them. One of their adult children suffered from emotional problems, and Paul's father had been living with them since his heart attack a few years before. Between their careers, their children, and caring for Paul's father, they simply didn't focus on what was happening to them. They were eating the same low-fat balanced diet they had for years, yet after Paul's father died, they realized they'd each gained about fifteen pounds and, for the first time in their lives, really began feeling their age.

"We just couldn't bear the thought of everything going downhill like that," Simone told me. "All of our lives we'd taken such good care of ourselves. I think what surprised me was how just a few years of dealing with a major life crisis had such an effect on us. Paul and I looked around and thought: We're not going to live forever either, but it doesn't have to be all downhill from here. Let's make it the best that we can, for ourselves and for our children."

After about a year of following a moderately intense exercise schedule that called for three aerobic sessions a week, plus some weight training for Simone, they'd both trimmed down and really firmed up. The most amazing progress was in their body-fat percentages. Simone dropped from 35 percent to 20 percent, and Paul from 28 percent to 18 percent. In the process, they improved their cardiovascular fitness and revved up their metabolism. Now they had the edge.

As you work toward your fitness goals, you'll probably want to learn how much further you can go to improve your health. Here's a look at how to control the things we can and learn to live with those we can't.

ALL ABOUT BODY FAT

Cellulite: It's Not All Just in Your Head

Some scientists and physicians insist there's no such thing as cellulite, yet every time about 90 percent of women look in the mirror, there it is: dimpled patches of skin that look as if they were stuffed with cottage cheese. So, yes, there is such a thing as cellulite, and it is fat. Contrary to fashion magazines and ads for miracle cures, however, cellulite is not really different from "regular" fat. The telltale difference—those little lumps and dents—is the result of the physical relationship between the skin and the fat directly beneath it. Beneath your skin lie vertical bands of fibrous tissue. When fat gets deposited in the areas in between them, these spots plump like little pillows while the "lines" of fibrous tissue create the "valleys." The greater the amount of fat, the "lumpier" the skin.

Cellulite is a perfectly normal, common, and even necessary (for successful child-bearing and nursing) component of the healthy female body. There are steps you can take to diminish the presence of cellulite, but despite cellulite-busting claims made on behalf of creams, massage, supplements, herbs, and liposuction, you will never totally banish it. Heredity (if your mother has cellulite, you probably do too), leading a seden-tary life, and eating a high-fat diet make cellulite more likely, but none of these factors alone causes it. That's why you can't fight cellulite on a single "front."

Fat, Toxins, and Weight Loss

When our bodies are exposed to toxins—pesticides and pollutants in our food, water, and air—they attempt to flush them through our systems. Our kidneys, livers, and other organs are constantly working to eliminate waste products and other substances from our bodies through urination, defecation, sweating, and breathing. Most of the time, we're fairly successful at keeping our internal "environments" clean, but when our bodies are overloaded by a number of environmental assaults or we fail to rid our-selves of them, they are deposited in our fat cells.

When we begin burning stored fat through diet, exercise, or a combination of the two, these heretofore "contained" toxins enter our bloodstreams and find new homes in other organs and tissues. The fatigue, headache, and overall crummy feeling most of us associate with losing weight is the result of the sudden surge in "loose" toxins. Since nothing we do to burn fat can also "burn" toxins, it's important to do all you can to help your body eliminate them as quickly as possible.

What Works: A Combination of Approaches

There is a lot you can do to lose fat and to minimize cellulite to the point where it's barely noticeable. One very effective dietary approach involves increasing your intake of so-called flushing foods, foods that attract toxins and/or move through the digestive system quickly and carry toxins out with them. Flushing foods include oil (2 table-spoons of flaxseed oil a day), rice and whole grains, vegetables, pineapple, apples, figs, berries, and citrus fruits. And don't forget eight to ten glasses of water every day.

The key is to do a combination of things:

- **EAT A LOW-FAT DIET.** How low do you go? The American Heart Association recommends that 30 percent or less of your daily calories come from fat, while some other experts think 10 percent is more conducive to good health. The majority opinion reflects a middle ground, no more than 20 percent of calories from fat.

- **LOWER YOUR OVERALL BODY FAT THROUGH DIET AND AN EXERCISE PROGRAM THAT TONES THE UNDERLYING MUSCLES.** In other words, fat-burning aerobics can't do the job alone. You also need resistance training to increase muscle tone.

- **GET A MASSAGE.** An experienced masseuse can manually break up the bands of tissue that contribute to the appearance of cellulite. You can also massage yourself using a loofah or a body brush (no need to invest in fancy anticellulite devices).

What Doesn't Work

- **LIPOSUCTION.** Who hasn't dreamed of having that excess fat "vacuumed" out once and for all? Who doesn't secretly thrill to the idea of lying down on a doctor's table and getting up a short time later magically transformed? It sounds too good to be true, and for cellulite, it essentially is. The trouble is, while liposuction does remove fat cells, it does nothing to eliminate the physical structure of the skin and the subcutaneous fat. A newer technique called superficial liposuctioning can improve the appearance up to 50 percent. For women who are not excessively overweight, liposuction can actually make the dimpling worse.

- **TOPICAL CREAMS, NUTRITIONAL SUPPLEMENTS AND PILLS, NEW TREATMENTS.** Don't waste your money. These simply do not work.

Remember: Most of us will have cellulite sooner or later. You may do everything possible outlined above and find yourself in a state of optimal health and still have some cellulite. If you lose this battle, remind yourself of what your most venerable opponent, Mother Nature, has on her side: millions of years of evolution. Once you're satisfied you've done all that you can to reduce cellulite, accept how you look and move on. There is more to life than firm thighs, and the time you may devote to chasing an unrealistic goal could be better spent changing something you really can.

CELLULITE AND MOTHERHOOD

You don't have to have borne and nursed children to develop cellulite, but doing so increases the amount you have. The reason is that during pregnancy, a woman's body stores fat in preparation for nursing. A woman's fat cells release more fat during lactation than at any other time, which suggests that even unwanted fat has a biological purpose.

FLAX FACTS

The seed of the blue-flowering flax plant has been an important food since at least 5000 B.C. In the eighth century, Charlemagne believed flaxseed so crucial to his nation's health that he created special legislation regarding its consumption. Today, flaxseed is far more commonly used in Europe and in Canada than it is here in the United States. But that may be about to change.

What Is It?

Flaxseed is emerging as a nutritional superstar, and deservedly so. It consists of 28 percent fiber and 20 percent protein, but the real magic lies in its 41 percent fat, because only 9 percent of it is saturated. The other 91 percent is divided between monounsaturated fat (18 percent) and polyunsaturated fat (73 percent). But it gets even better. The polyunsaturated fat is a combination of 57 percent omega-3 and 16 percent omega-6, a ratio of 3:1, so including flaxseed and flaxseed oil in your diet may help you achieve a healthier proportion between the omega oils; ideally, it should be 1 (omega-3) to 1 (omega-6). (See "What Are EFAs?," page 142.) In addition, flaxseed also contains potassium (seven times that of a banana, ounce for ounce) and small amounts of magnesium, iron, copper, and zinc. Flaxseed is rich in lignans, a form of phytoestrogens that show promise in the prevention of hormone-dependent cancers, such as breast cancer.

Flax and Weight Loss

Some fat is essential to health, but there is good fat and there is bad fat (see "Fat at a Glance," page 144). Most of us eat far too much fat, and most of that fat is saturated, hydrogenated, or trans fat—the worst kind. It may take a bit of "diet myth reprogramming" to believe this, but it's true. The right amount of the right kind of fat can help you lose weight, and flaxseed oil is that fat. Its omega-3 and omega-6 fatty acids stimulate the metabolism of fat. Consuming as little as 1 to 2 tablespoons of flaxseed oil a day can eliminate your craving for other fats. How so? Interestingly, a deficiency in omega-3 fat will cue a craving for any kind of fat. You might say you're craving the wrong fats because you're not getting enough of the right ones.

How to Put More Flaxseed in Your Diet

If you're embarking on a major lifestyle change—trying to lose weight, diminish cellulite and other body fat, or change your eating habits—don't even start without a bottle of flaxseed oil in the fridge. Try a tablespoon once or twice a day, but don't forget that this is a substitution for other fats in your diet, not an addition to them. Flaxseed oil contains the same 100 calories per tablespoon as other vegetable, nut, and seed oils. If you can take it straight, do so. Otherwise, mix it into your salad dressing, drizzle it on grilled vegetables, or chase it with a big glass of juice.

Eating whole or milled flaxseed gives you the benefit of its protein, fiber, and vitamin content. Whole or milled flaxseed can be added to batters for cakes, cookies, breads, pancakes, and muffins. You can use a mixture of milled flaxseed to replace oil or shortening in some recipes. For every half cup of oil, margarine, butter, or shortening, use 1½ cups milled flaxseed. The substitution will drastically lower the amount of saturated fat in the recipe, though baked foods may brown a little more quickly. People who don't eat eggs might experiment with replacing each egg called for in batter recipes with a mixture of 1 tablespoon of milled flaxseed and 3 tablespoons of water. Let stand for a couple minutes, then add to the mix. The resulting texture will be smaller in volume and chewier. Perhaps one day we'll have access to omega-3 eggs, which are now available in Canada. These eggs, produced by hens fed flaxseed-enriched feed, contain up to twelve times the omega-3 fats of regular eggs.

TWO EXERCISES TO BETTER SEX

We all know that sex is a physical activity, but we don't always appreciate how much we can improve our performance, endurance, and pleasure by toning specific muscle groups, particularly in the buttocks, pelvis, and back. We also know that a lot of how we feel about sex is in our minds, and nothing makes you feel sexier and more attractive than having strong body confidence.

The Superman Lift

This exercise strengthens your back and your buttocks.

1. Lie on your stomach with your arms extended in front of you, shoulder-width apart (think of Superman in flight). Keep your head aligned with your spine and your toes pointed down.

2. Take a deep breath. As you exhale, lift your left leg in a controlled motion, toes pointed, back straight, your hip bones still touching the floor. Don't stop until you can't go any higher without bending your knee.

3. Take a deep breath. As you inhale, lower your leg in a slow, controlled movement.

4. Alternate legs for a total of two sets of eight reps.

Lower-Body Toner

This exercise has two benefits: It increases your pelvic range of motion, and it also teaches you how to isolate the muscles of your pelvis so that you can move your pelvis without moving the rest of your body.

1. Sit with knees bent, hands and feet flat on the floor, with your fingers pointing behind you.

2. With your arms, raise your lower body a few inches off the floor.

3. Twist your right hip and pelvic region down; this will cause your left side to rise slightly. Then do the same on your opposite side.

4. Slowly, do ten reps. Lower your body to the floor and relax.

APHRODISIACS IN YOUR PANTRY?

For a long time, scientists scoffed at the old wives' tales surrounding man's—and woman's—quest for the mystical food or drink with the power to spark sexual attraction and enhance sexual performance. Now that the laboratory's unveiled the chemical secrets of these long-purported love-enhancing foods, it seems those old wives—not to mention their old husbands—might have been a little more hip than we thought. True, there is no such thing as a guaranteed aphrodisiac in the sense of a "love potion." But sex is a physical and emotional experience deeply intertwined with other pleasurable experiences, including eating and drinking. Try setting the mood with any of these:

- **CELERY AND CELERIAC (CELERY ROOT)** contain androsterone, a male hormone whose scent women find attractive. All parts of the celery plant are considered to have aphrodisiac qualities, especially the seeds, which can be added to salad dressings and salads.

- **CHOCOLATE** contains phenylethylamine (PEA), which can prompt a rise in endorphins—the "feel good" neurochemicals—and caffeine, which can make you feel more alert and focused. The legendary lover Casanova was a chocoholic, and it's probably no coincidence that more chocolate is sold on Valentine's Day than any other.

- **OYSTERS**—like the majority of alleged aphrodisiacs—earned part of their reputation at least on their looks. Basically, any food that resembled genitalia was deemed to possess stimulating power (this explains the appeal of asparagus and bananas, tomatoes, cherries, and peaches—do you see a pattern here?), and raw oysters fit this role nicely. However, there's more to oysters than just their look, feel, and smell. Ounce for ounce, oysters contain more of the mineral zinc than any other food. And deficiencies in zinc have been found to cause impotence, decreased testosterone levels, and low sperm counts. Zinc also calms the nerves, which may help set the mood.

- **PINE NUTS (PIGNOLIA),** a key ingredient in pesto sauce, is another zinc-rich food that's been hailed for its aphrodisiac qualities since ancient times.

SCENTS TO SEND YOU

We spend billions every year on perfumes and colognes, in part because we believe (even subconsciously) the advertisers' claims that manufactured scents enhance our sex appeal. But do they? Recent research suggests that, contrary to what their manufacturers would like us to believe, perfume, cologne, and aftershave are actually a turnoff. This is particularly true for women. That may be because they mask the smell of natural body chemicals that do turn us on: the elusive but undeniably powerful pheromones.

Of course, we each have individual preferences, but here's what we know about the scents that really turn us on. Men respond to the scent of cinnamon, roast meat, pizza, chocolate, vanilla, strawberry (so that's how they came up with Neapolitan ice cream!), and peppermint. Among the spice scents with long aphrodisiac traditions that men respond to favorably are ginger, clove, coriander, and nutmeg. In one study, exposure to some of these scents increased penile blood flow by 40 percent. Women were found to favor the vanilla-ish, licorice scent of Good & Plenty candy. Interestingly, fennel (which has a licorice-like smell) was considered an aphrodisiac as far back as 1600 B.C. Earlier this century in rural areas of this country, women prepared for courtin' with strategically placed dabs of vanilla extract. It seems our foremothers knew how to get things cooking, and not just on the stove.

Moving from the kitchen to the garden, the scents that cast a spell on both men and women seem to be jasmine (Cleopatra's favorite), sandalwood, neroli (from oranges), ylang-ylang, lily, lilac, and tuberose.

HOW SEX KEEPS WOMEN AND MEN HEALTHY

Sexual activity is good for your health. An orgasm burns over 200 calories, and provides an intense, if brief, cardiovascular miniworkout. Sexual excitement prompts the release of three important hormones: estrogen and testosterone, which boost the immune system, and DHEA, which helps reduce blood cholesterol and body fat.

BANISH PMS WITH NUTRITION

Premenstrual syndrome, which affects an estimated 40 to 60 percent of women of childbearing age—can encompass any one of dozens of cyclical physical and emotional changes. Among the most common complaints are breast tenderness, headache, bloating, pelvic pain, weight gain, joint swelling, and a wide range of emotional changes: nervousness, anxiety, depression, mood swings, anger, difficulty focusing, and lack of interest in usual activities.

Common as it is, every woman's PMS is unique in terms of symptoms, timing, and severity. Even though PMS was first identified in the 1930s, it was not studied seriously until the 1980s. Since then, it has been the subject of countless studies. For most women, preventing or relieving symptoms is usually a case of trial and error. What works for one woman doesn't necessarily work for another. While the dramatic hormonal changes that define the menstrual cycle are the "ground zero" of PMS, why each woman's body responds to those changes is not so clear. One thing we do know is that for millions of PMS sufferers, dietary changes can be very effective. An important 1998 controlled study in which half the women received 1,200 milligrams of calcium and the other half got a placebo demonstrated a 54 percent reduction in symptoms. In light of these findings, it's worth considering whether the real culprit in PMS is the hormonal fluctuations (for example, an increase in estrogen production) or the fact that so many of us fail to support our bodies nutritionally to tolerate those changes. After all, we all should be getting at least 1,000 milligrams of calcium a day, yet more than 90 percent of us fail to get even *half* that. Maybe PMS isn't such a mystery after all.

While there isn't yet a one-size-fits-all solution to PMS, we know enough that many of us can easily custom-tailor an anti-PMS plan based on exercise, nutrition, and lifestyle changes. The even better news is that anything you do to block or alleviate PMS will have myriad other health benefits, as you'll see below.

If you experience PMS symptoms that are debilitating or severe, see your physician to rule out the possibility that your symptoms are not indicative of another, possibly more serious, condition or one that would respond to other forms of treatment.

How to Block PMS

Except in rare cases, PMS is not necessarily inevitable. While some symptoms might be less responsive to changes in lifestyle and nutrition (for example, migraine headaches), others—such as bloating, breast tenderness, and food cravings—can be dramatically reduced, even eliminated. Again, for most women, this is a process of trial and error. Be patient; it may take three or four cycles before you see symptom relief. Also note, over one hundred different symptoms now fall under the heading *PMS*. While the chart below specifically addresses only the most common, consider trying these suggestions for other symptoms.

PMS: WHAT HELPS

BE SURE YOU GET ENOUGH . . .	TO RELIEVE . . .	BECAUSE . . .
vitamin B complex	*cramps, depression, irritability, mood swings, water retention, and weight gain*	*they help metabolize estrogen.*
vitamin C	*breast tenderness, constipation, water retention, and weight gain*	*it helps metabolize estrogen.*
calcium	*cramps and mood swings*	*it helps relax muscle tissue and improves nerve-impulse transmission.*
complex-carbohydrate foods (whole grains, rice, and pasta)	*cramps, depression, irritability, and mood swings*	*they help raise serotonin levels and short-circuit food cravings.*
vitamin E	*breast tenderness, cramps, fatigue, headache, and insomnia*	*it helps metabolize estrogen.*
magnesium	*cramps and mood swings*	*it works with calcium and helps metabolize estrogen.*
soy products (soybeans, tofu, tempeh, soy cheeses, and other foods)	*breast tenderness and cramps*	*the phytoestrogens in soy reduce the impact of natural estrogen on cells.*

PMS: WHAT HELPS

BE SURE YOU GET ENOUGH . . .	TO RELIEVE . . .	BECAUSE . . . *(continued)*
water, eight to ten glasses a day	*constipation, water retention, and weight gain*	*paradoxically, it's too little water that causes water retention, not too much. (See "The Real Water Cure," page 22.)*

What Exacerbates PMS

- **ALCOHOL.** It takes less than a single drink to cause a dramatic drop in blood sugar that can last up to seventy-two hours, contributing to depression, fatigue, headache, insomnia, and mood swings.

- **CAFFEINE.** In some women, caffeine seems to exacerbate some PMS symptoms, particularly irritability and breast tenderness. There are several theories as to why this might be so, but there is persuasive anecdotal evidence to support at least giving up caffeine from all food sources (coffee, tea, chocolate, soft drinks) on a trial basis for about three months.

- **DAIRY PRODUCTS.** Again, the evidence is largely anecdotal but compelling, though no one is exactly sure how dairy products affect PMS. One theory is that some of us are extremely sensitive to the antibiotics and hormones most dairy products contain. There are people who believe that humans simply were not intended to ingest the milk of any species other than their own, and that PMS symptoms are one of a wide range of dairy-induced "allergic reactions." You should know within a month or two after quitting dairy if this is your problem.

- **SALT.** Excess salt increases water retention.

- **SUGAR.** Eating too much sugar creates swings in your blood-sugar level and often takes the place of more nutritious foods you could be eating instead, such as complex carbohydrates, fresh fruits and vegetables, and high-quality, low-fat protein. One study found that PMS sufferers consumed over two and a half times the sugar other women did.

What Else Alleviates PMS Symptoms?

Studies have found that regular aerobic exercise, relaxation, stress reduction, and a few minutes in the sun each day (if possible) can all help. If breast tenderness is a problem, check your bra. Tight bras—particularly those with underwires—can block circulation of both blood and lymph fluid, resulting in congestion and exacerbation of your discomfort. Try switching to a well-fitting soft-cup or sports bra when you can.

YOU CAN AVOID MIDDLE-AGE SPREAD

This will probably alarm you: Between the ages of twenty-five and fifty-five, the average American will gain 1 pound per year. That's 30 extra, unhealthy, and unwanted pounds simply because we eat too much of the wrong foods and don't exercise enough. And women get a double whammy when menopause hits, as the effects of declining estrogen on metabolism and fat-distribution patterns disrupt the fat-to-lean ratio. Until recently, we simply resigned ourselves to the inevitable, telling ourselves that our metabolism was slowing with age and believing there was nothing we could do. It's time to change your thinking on this, whether you're middle-aged right now or plan to be anytime in the future.

What We Now Know About Middle-Age Spread

First, it's not inevitable, and it's not beyond your control. Second, and more important, middle-age spread signals increased risk for heart disease, diabetes, and some forms of cancer. For women, middle-age spread is the result of changes in behavior, which we can change, and changes in our bodies, which we cannot prevent but which we can learn to compensate for. Generally speaking, as we grow older, we become less active. In a cruel twist, the less active we are, the more slowly our body burns calories even when we're resting. We compound the problem when we allow our muscle mass to decline, because when we rest, muscle tissue requires more energy to simply exist than fat tissue. Sedentary women lose a half pound of muscle mass a year just by doing nothing. The resulting drop in the resting metabolic rate may explain why even though you're eating the same way you did ten years ago and not exercising any less, the pounds have started creeping on.

Making women even more susceptible to middle-age spread are the hormonal changes they experience with age. When we're premenopausal and menstruating regularly, our bodies burn up 15,000 to 20,000 calories every year as our metabolic rates rise in the two weeks preceding menstruation. We're happily unaware of how efficiently our bodies keep these potential 4½ to 6 pounds at bay until it stops.

With encroaching menopause, not only do we burn fewer calories, but our bodies start to handle the calories and fat distribution differently than they did before. European researchers discovered that an enzyme called lipoprotein lipase, which controls fat-cell growth, may be rendered less active by the presence of estrogen. When estrogen levels begin their gradual decline, the lipoprotein lipase causes more fat to be deposited in the middle. Another study looked at SHBG (sex-hormone-binding globulin), a molecule that attaches to and disables the small amounts of testosterone our bodies produce. SHBG levels decline as estrogen goes down, so that not only are women producing a larger proportion of testosterone than they were before menopause, but without SHBG to counter it, the testosterone has a greater effect. The most obvious is the tendency to accumulate body fat in the upper body, in a more male-type pattern. This is why even women who maintain the same body weight they had in their late teens or early twenties will notice that their shape has changed: The waistline isn't as well defined, if it's there at all.

What Won't Work

- **TRYING TO RECAPTURE A SLIMMER YOU THROUGH DIET ALONE.** Simply losing weight will not stop the spread permanently. Without exercise you may lose some fat, but you will also lose muscle, and less muscle means a lower resting-metabolism rate. Chances are, whatever you do lose through diet alone will eventually return, and repeat dieting may prompt your body to further slow your metabolism to protect you from starving. (Your metabolism has no way of understanding what a diet is.)

- **STRIVING FOR THE FAT-TO-MUSCLE RATIO OF YOUR YOUNGER YEARS.** While you can do much through exercise and diet to reduce the impact of your postmenopausal body's tendency to store fat in the midsection, you cannot eliminate it entirely. Postmenopausal women who did not exercise had over double the fat mass as postmenopausal women who exercised regularly.

What Helps

- **WEIGHT-BEARING EXERCISE** builds muscle and bone mass, both important for continued health after menopause.

- **AEROBIC EXERCISE** helps burn up the calories your resting metabolism can't quite handle, and it raises your metabolic rate.

- **EATING SENSIBLY,** with the realization that you are not burning calories the way you used to.

And Even If Menopause Seems a Long Time Away . . .

Start changing your habits—and improving your health—right now. Menopause does not occur overnight. It's a gradual process that begins imperceptibly years before you experience any of the telltale symptoms. While it's impossible to predict how anyone will respond to this important change, you can do a lot today to improve your chances of continued health and well-being in your postmenopausal years.

YOU'RE NEVER TOO YOUNG TO THINK ABOUT ARTHRITIS

Aging Baby Boomers may be surprised to find themselves part of what experts are calling a future arthritis epidemic. In the next two decades, nearly 20 percent of the population (the majority of them women) will have arthritis or another rheumatic condition. Even now, it is the leading cause of disability. The term *arthritis* encompasses over a hundred different diseases that affect the joints. The most common form is osteoarthritis, where the wear and tear of living results in a painful breakdown of cartilage, the dense, spongy protein that cushions the joints and keeps bones (for instance, in the knee, spine, and wrist) from rubbing against each other. Another form, rheumatoid arthritis, is actually an autoimmune disease, in which the immune system indiscriminately "attacks" and provokes inflammation in joints, cartilage, and bone.

Reducing the Risk of Osteoarthritis

Until recently, arthritis has been considered inevitable, and earlier medical wisdom advocated practices—such as avoiding physical exercise—that we now know actually make the condition worse. While the causes of rheumatoid arthritis are still unclear, there is a lot you can do now to reduce your risk of developing osteoarthritis.

- **EXERCISE REGULARLY AND PROPERLY.** Don't overuse or abuse your body, and pay particular attention to those areas most vulnerable to injury and arthritis: the knee, shoulder, wrist, and back.

- **IF YOU DEVELOP PERSISTENT PAIN, SEE AN ORTHOPEDIST IMMEDIATELY.** A specialist can make the right diagnosis and prescribe exercises or physical therapy to prevent further damage. Just by increasing your awareness of movements you should avoid, you can avoid exacerbating the damage.

- **AVOID DOING THINGS THAT STRESS OR DAMAGE VULNERABLE, ARTHRITIS-PRONE AREAS.** So much of this is simple common sense, but it bears repeating. Simple things such as lifting heavy objects properly, setting up your work space for maximum ergonomic comfort, and not wearing high heels go a long way in preventing the stress or injury that opens the door to osteoarthritis.

Coping with Osteoarthritis

If you have osteoarthritis, there's a lot you can do. While you can't turn back the clock and undo the damage that has been done, you can help yourself to feel better now.

- **NUTRITIONAL SUPPLEMENTS.** Probably the hottest news for arthritis sufferers is that about half of those who try a combination of the supplements glucosamine (500 mg. three times a day) and chondroitin sulfate (500 mg. three times a day) claim to see a decrease in pain and stiffness. You should know that no major studies have been done in this. The few done in Europe were promising, and though they seem safe for short-term use, no one has determined the effects of long-term use. The Arthritis Foundation does not endorse their use.

- **GENERAL DIET GUIDELINES.** Eat a balanced diet high in antioxidants and bioflavonoids, low in fat and trans-fatty acids (which can encourage inflammation). Bioflavonoids are high in citrus, green tea, berries, onions, and any fruit that contains a pit.

- **EXERCISE.** Yoga, Arthritis Foundation–approved water exercise classes, tai chi, and other low-impact activities are highly recommended. Moderate weight-bearing exercise, such as walking, biking, swimming, and low-impact aerobics, can build bones and the muscles around your damaged joint, for added support. Just be sure to check with your doctor before you begin a program.

- **PAMPER YOURSELF.** Beyond medications to reduce pain and inflammation, you can help yourself with acupressure, hydrotherapy (moist heat packs or a dip in a hot tub, Jacuzzi, or pool with a water temperature of at least 85 degrees F.), aromatherapy baths (rosemary or chamomile oil), massage, relaxation and meditation, and acupuncture.

SAVE YOUR SKIN—AND POSSIBLY YOUR LIFE

Nothing damages and ages your skin like the sun. By now, you'd think we'd have all gotten the message, but apparently even vanity and visions of creased leathery skin can't compete with the immediate longing for the perfect tan. Equally disturbing is the fact that millions of us who think we're doing everything to save our skins are actually overlooking crucial precautions. And most recently, the news that sunscreens and sunblocks may not guard against melanoma, the most deadly form of skin cancer, has some people breaking out the suntan oil and the aluminum reflectors again.

UVA and UVB, SPF and PABA—it can be confusing. But learn and follow these basics and you'll be sitting pretty—forever.

- **CHANGE YOUR ATTITUDE.** Sunscreens and sunblocks do not "prevent" cancer; they simply lower your risk by limiting your exposure to cancer-causing rays. For people with a genetic susceptibility to melanoma, they may not help at all. Don't assume that it's ever "safe" to be out in the sun.

- **IF YOU HAVE SKIN, YOU'RE AT RISK FOR SKIN CANCER, NO MATTER WHAT YOUR AGE, NATIONALITY, SKIN COLOR, HAIR COLOR, OR EYE COLOR.** Yes, blondes and redheads, and people with fair skin and blue or green eyes do have a higher incidence of skin cancer. However, people with dark skins—including African Americans—do develop skin cancer.

- **EVERYONE SHOULD WEAR SUNSCREEN, EVERY DAY.** The American Academy of Dermatology and the Skin Cancer Foundation recommend that everyone wear sunscreen with at least an SPF (sun protection factor) of 15.

- **THERE'S NO SUCH THING AS A "SAFE" TIME TO SUN.** You can reduce your exposure to the sun's harmful ultraviolet rays by over half simply by staying out of the sun from 10:00 A.M. to 4:00 P.M. (11:00 A.M. and 5:00 P.M. Daylight Savings Time), when the sun's UVB rays (those that cause sunburn) are the harshest. (This applies to North America; the sun is stronger as you move closer to the equator.) That doesn't mean, however, that the rays you're exposed to at other times are not harmful. The UVA rays are strongest early in the morning and later in the afternoon, and while they don't cause sunburn, they are responsible for the changes that result in aging. Only sunblocks and sunscreens of SPF 15 or higher can block UVA rays.

- **THERE IS NO SUCH THING AS A "SAFE" SEASON.** Too many people are "sun conscious" during spring and summer, then toss the sunscreen in the closet until next Memorial Day. Don't! The sun may be farther away, but its ultraviolet rays are bouncing all around us, reflected from the ground, concrete, sand, water, ice, and snow. (This is why a beach umbrella or wide-brimmed hat cannot afford complete protection.)

- **THERE IS NO SUCH THING AS "SAFE" WEATHER.** Eighty percent of ultraviolet rays penetrate clouds, haze, fog, and rain.

- **USE THE MOST EFFECTIVE SUNBLOCK AND/OR SUNSCREEN YOU CAN FIND.** Sunblocks completely deflect ultraviolet rays. They are opaque, so you can't use them every day, but they provide excellent protection for those easily burned lips, earlobes, and nose. Zinc oxide and titanium dioxide are the two most effective active ingredients.

Sunscreens come in a dizzying array of formulations and SPFs. Here's all you need to know:

1. Look for a sunscreen that blocks both UVB and UVA. And don't assume yours does unless the label specifically states that it does. Generally, the SPF applies only to UVB protection.

2. Wear the highest SPF you can every day. The higher the SPF rating, the more UVA it will screen. SPFs range from 2 (useless) to 50.

3. Buy the sunscreen with the most effective active ingredients. Look for:

   PABA or benzophenone (the two most effective)
   oxybenzone
   sulisobenzone
   Parsol 1789, or butyl methoxydibenzoylmenthane, or avobenzone
   titanium dioxide
   zinc oxide

4. If you find that you're sensitive to a particular sunscreen, don't give up. Try another with different active ingredients. Some people are allergic to PABA.

5. Avoid oil and gel sunscreens; they're not as effective as lotions and creams.

6. Do not apply sunscreen or sunblock around your eyes. The skin there is extremely sensitive, and chemicals in sunscreens are very irritating to the eye itself. Because many of these sunscreens are water resistant or waterproof, they are difficult to rinse away once they get into your eyes. Instead, wear sunglasses that block UV rays to cover the area around your eyes.

7. Apply sunscreen or sunblock at least twenty minutes before going out into the sun. Even "waterproof" or "water resistant" products are washed away by water and sweat or rubbed away through normal "wear." Reapply thoroughly as necessary.

8. Apply sunscreen everywhere, then cover up. Ultraviolet rays can penetrate light summer clothing. Nine out of ten skin cancers develop on areas of the body rarely or never exposed to the sun. Contrary to popular belief, light clothing does not "reflect" the sun's rays back—it actually conducts them toward the skin.

SUNBURN HELP FROM THE KITCHEN

Used tea bags can help relieve the pain of sunburn. After the tea bag has steeped and cooled, gently dab it on sunburned areas. The tannic acid will reduce inflammation. A long soak in a lukewarm bath that contains 1 to 2 cups of dry oatmeal will also moisturize and soothe sunburned skin.

IMPROVE YOUR HEALTH IN TWENTY MINUTES: QUIT SMOKING

Sounds too good to be true, doesn't it? But it's a fact: Within minutes of putting out that last cigarette, your body begins to undergo a series of changes that, over time, effectively undo much of the damage smoking has inflicted.

Research reveals that smoking is more dangerous and has more far-reaching effects than first believed. Because smoking diminishes blood flow through the capillary veins, it makes wounds slower to heal and the spinal discs that cushion the vertebrae stiffen. The chemicals in smoke not only ruin skin, discolor nails, and yellow teeth, they also compromise the stomach's ability to protect itself from stomach acid. Nicotine is now believed to exacerbate PMS, and smokers contract more colds and experience more dramatic allergy symptoms than nonsmokers.

Of course, no one said quitting was easy. While some folks can drop the habit cold turkey, most of us need a couple of tries and the help of a support group and a period of nicotine replacement therapy (such as the patch and nicotine gums). It's not always easy to deny the moment's cravings for a potentially longer and healthier life somewhere in the distant future. As they say, you've got to take it one day at a time. But, as the old song says and as research now reveals: What a difference a day makes!

WHAT HAPPENS AFTER YOU QUIT SMOKING

20 minutes after you quit . . .	Your blood pressure drops to normal. Your pulse rate drops to normal.
8 hours after you quit . . .	Your blood oxygen level increases to normal.
24 hours after you quit . . .	Your chance of suffering a heart attack decreases.
48 hours after you quit . . .	Your ability to smell and taste is enhanced. You find it easier to walk.
2 weeks to 3 months after you quit . . .	Your lung function—your lungs' ability to efficiently deliver oxygen to your heart and throughout your body—increases up to 30 percent. PMS symptoms—which are exacerbated by nicotine—become less severe.
1 to 9 months after you quit . . .	You experience shortness of breath less often.
1 year after you quit . . .	Your risk of coronary artery disease is half what it was while you were still smoking. You will experience half as many colds and allergy attacks. Crow's feet–type facial wrinkles will be less prominent.

HOW TO LOWER YOUR RISK OF BREAST CANCER

No one can say for certain what your risk of developing breast cancer is. Like all other cancers, breast cancer is a complex disease whose source is rarely clear and may actually be the result of several factors. While no one knows how to "prevent" breast cancer, there is a tremendous, ever-growing body of research on what you can do to cut your risk.

There is little we can do to alter most of our other risk factors (such as how many years we menstruate, how many children we have and when, whether or not we breast-feed, and so on). Only a very small percentage of us are genetically predisposed to develop breast cancer. Even those people who face an increased risk, based on genetic testing, are encouraged to adopt risk-reducing lifestyle habits. Since 75 percent of breast malignancies occur in women over fifty, and cancer is a disease of aging, you may have years, even decades, to make these positive habits part of your life.

If you are concerned about breast cancer, you should know that this is a disease where misinformation and speculation run rampant. A classic case: the oft-quoted statistic that one in nine (or eight) women will develop breast cancer in her lifetime. In fact, the chances are one in nine *only if* you live to be eighty-five or older. This is not to say that we shouldn't be concerned about breast cancer; we should. But spending a lot of money on unproven supplements, megadoses of vitamins and minerals, and making bizarre dietary changes of little or no proven benefit may be misguided. There are four recognized lifestyle risk factors for breast cancer: severe obesity, sedentary lifestyle, excessive alcohol consumption, and a high-fat diet. (It is beyond the scope of this book to discuss medical issues involving hormone replacement therapy.) These are the effective, proven steps we can easily take today and every day:

- **EXERCISE.** Four hours of exercise each week can cut your risk by 37 percent.

- **LOSE THE FAT.** Being 40 percent or more heavier than your ideal weight increases your risk because the more body fat you carry, the more estrogen your cells are exposed to. And estrogen is a culprit in breast cancer development.

- **AVOID ALCOHOL.** A number of large studies have found an association between consuming alcohol in excess of three drinks per week and an increased incidence of breast cancer. In one, women who had three to nine drinks a week had a 30 percent increase in risk; anything more than that doubled the risk to 60 percent.

- **EAT A LOW-FAT, HIGH-FIBER, FRUIT-AND-VEGGIE-RICH DIET.** What constitutes "low fat" for purposes of cancer prevention is an area of some controversy. There is evidence that only diets that allow 20 percent *or less* of their daily calories to come from fat will make a difference. The fat you do eat should be monounsaturated and include the polyunsaturated omega-3, which has been proved to inhibit breast cancer cells. (See "Fat: Unlocking the Right

Combination," page 141.) Since there is some evidence that fiber binds estrogen and hastens its elimination, try to get 25 to 30 grams of fiber a day. Finally, eat low on the food chain: less meat, more complex carbohydrates, fruits, and vegetables. Fruits and vegetables still remain the best source of antioxidants, phytochemicals, flavonoids, indoles, isoflavones, lignans, and other chemicals that have demonstrated a measurable ability to inhibit cancer-cell development and growth. (See "Carbohydrates: The Best Sources of Anticancer Chemicals," page 148.)

Epilogue

I hope that you've reached the end of this book convinced that fitness is within your grasp. Because it is. In the many years I've been teaching about fitness and health, I've probably seen someone very much like you. People who have trouble cultivating a lifestyle where fit can happen tend to believe that their relationship to their bodies is a problem for which someone, *somewhere,* has the solution. The truth is, no one has "the" key. What works is different for everyone. If you wait around for a single answer to your fitness dilemma, you'll be waiting forever, and in vain.

When fit happens, it happens because of what we do *for* ourselves, not in spite of what we do *to* ourselves. It's not the product of an intensive two-month exercise regimen or a few weeks on a restrictive diet. Fitness isn't something that comes in a kit or falls from the sky complete and ready to run. It's something that you have to build, brick by brick. And unless you're a fitness or health professional, the pursuit of fitness will probably never become a lifestyle for you. Realistically, you have to make room for it within the confines and limitations of the lifestyle you already have. I've tried to demonstrate how doing that is as simple as replacing bad habits with good ones, making a handful of wiser choices at the market, and opting to reallocate three half hours of television time each week to physical movement.

If I've done nothing else with this book, I hope I've shown you how the situations we tend to view as roadblocks to fitness can be avoided simply and easily if we know where to find the detours around them. Those detours are paved with knowledge. Something as seemingly inconsequential as drinking enough water each day, or eating the right kind of food before a workout, can make all the difference, especially when you consider the domino effect that comes into play when we feel tired, out of sorts, and unequal to the task at hand. These emotions and attitudes are so often cited as the "reasons" for skipping that walk or going for that second helping, doesn't it make sense to give yourself every possible advantage throughout your day, no matter how small?

The human body is amazingly resilient. If you've changed anything as a result of this book, you've already noticed that extra bit of energy, that newfound glow. And the good news is that *you* did it. You made it happen. How you apply those small victories is up to you. Whether that means you don't start the next fad diet or you start training for a marathon isn't as important as the fact that you're now making practical, informed, and realistic decisions. And, remember, what you do now is just the beginning. Just as bad habits kick off and feed cycles of negative behavior, positive habits often jump-start more positive change. When you feel miserable, it's hard to think about exercise. But when you feel good and you've already lost a few pounds, it's hard to even consider not exercising.

Making fitness happen in your life is not only good for you, it's good for your family, too. I can't imagine a more enduring gift you can give your children than respect for their bodies and your example of sound, healthy habits to carry them through life.

Fit happens because you make it happen. Whatever changes you've made already, I urge you to keep growing and learning. Stay focused on your power to use information to help—not intimidate, mislead, or undermine—you. Become the only expert on you that you'll ever need. And let fit keep happening for you.

JOANIE GREGGAINS is one of America's favorite health and exercise personalities. Ever since she taught secondary school physical education in the early 1970s, Joanie has believed that fitness begins with knowledge. She became a popular, respected authority in the field in part through her long-running TV exercise program, *Morning Stretch* (since 1979), and her talk-radio show, *The Joanie Greggains Show,* on KGO Radio 810 AM in San Francisco since 1985. The producer of her television program, she has also written, choreographed, and starred in thirteen fitness videos and is the author of *Total Shape-Up*. Joanie has served on the President's Council for Physical Fitness and the California Governor's Council on Physical Fitness and Sports. She has received the Jaycees of America's Fitness Leader Award and holds multiple certifications for fitness training. She is co-owner of ProActive Fitness Center, a personal-training facility in Mill Valley, California, and is a popular motivational speaker and spokesperson. She lives in the Bay Area.

PATRICIA ROMANOWSKI is an award-winning editor and the coauthor of eighteen books, including three national best-sellers—Mary Wilson's *Dreamgirl: My Life as a Supreme;* Vanna White's *Vanna Speaks;* and La Toya Jackson's *La Toya*—and a best-selling trilogy of books on the psychic medium George Anderson, including *We Don't Die*. Other titles include Donny Osmond's *Life Is Just What You Make It: My Story So Far;* Teddy Pendergrass's *Truly Blessed;* M. Gary Neuman's *Helping Your Kids Cope with Divorce the Sandcastles Way;* and, with Joel Martin, *Love Beyond Life: The Healing Power of After-Death Communications*. She is an editor of both editions of *The Rolling Stone Encyclopedia of Rock & Roll* and coauthor of Otis Williams's *Temptations,* on which the popular NBC miniseries was based, and Annette Funicello's *A Dream Is a Wish Your Heart Makes: My Story*. She lives on Long Island with her husband, author Philip Bashe, and their son, Justin.